Clinical Oncology

J. W. Sweetenham BSc, MB, BS, MRCP
Senior Registrar, Cancer Research Campaign
Medical Oncology Unit, Southampton University Hospitals

F. R. Macbeth MA, DM, MRCP, FRCR
Consultant, Beatson Oncology Centre, Western Infirmary, Glasgow

G. M. Mead DM, MRCP
Consultant Medical Oncologist, Cancer Research Campaign
Medical Oncology Unit, Southampton University Hospitals

C. J. H. Williams DM, FRCP
Honorary Consultant Physician, Cancer Research Campaign
Medical Oncology Unit, Southampton University Hospitals

J. M. A. Whitehouse MA, MD, FRCP
Director, Cancer Research Campaign
Medical Oncology Unit, Southampton University Hospitals

Second edition

PRESENTED BY

Boehringer Ingelheim, Hospital Division
MANUFACTURERS OF BONEFOS® AND ORAMORPH®

Blackwell Scientific Publications
OXFORD LONDON EDINBURGH BOSTON
MELBOURNE PARIS BERLIN VIENNA

© 1989 by
Blackwell Scientific Publications
Editorial offices:
Osney Mead, Oxford OX2 0EL
25 John Street, London WC1N 2BL
23 Ainslie Place, Edinburgh EH3
  6AJ
238 Main Street, Cambridge
  Massachusetts 02142, USA
54 University Street, Carlton
  Victoria 3053, Australia

Other Editorial Offices:
Librairie Arnette SA
2, rue Casimir-Delavigne
75006 Paris
France

Blackwell Wissenschafts-Verlag
Meinekestrasse 4
D-1000 Berlin 15
Germany

Blackwell MZV
Feldgasse 13
A-1238 Wien
Austria

First published 1983
Second edition 1989
Reprinted 1993

Set by Times Graphics,
Singapore and printed and
bound in Great Britain at
The Alden Press, Oxford

DISTRIBUTORS

Marston Book Services Ltd
PO Box 87
Oxford OX2 0DT
(*Orders*: Tel: 0865-791155
          Fax: 0865-791927
          Telex: 837515)

USA
Blackwell Scientific Publications, Inc.
238 Main Street
Cambridge, MA 02142
(*Orders*: Tel: 800 759-6102
           617 876-7000)

Canada
Times Mirror Professional
Publishing, Ltd
130 Flaska Drive
Markham, Ontario L6G 1B8
(*Orders*: Tel: 800 268-4178
           416 470-6739)

Australia
Blackwell Scientific Publications
(Australia) Pty Ltd
54 University Street
Carlton, Victoria 3053
(*Orders*: Tel: 03 347-5552)

British Library
Cataloguing in Publication Data

Sweetenham, J. W.
  Clinical oncology—2nd ed.
  1. Man. Cancer. Therapy
  I. Title   II. Series
  616.99'406

ISBN 0-632-02449-6

Contents

Preface

The complexity of modern cancer management requires an increasing range of information to be readily available to those involved in the daily care of the cancer patient.

This book is not intended as an exhaustive guide but as a prompt to good management. The emphasis is therefore on the practical. As a pocket book it should be easy to carry and easy to use. It has been divided into sections for ease of reference with cross references where appropriate. Inevitably some managements cannot be standardized and those listed are only intended as a guide. A new section is concerned with radiotherapy and deals with the management of some problems which may be treated by radiotherapy and also some common side-effects of treatment.

List of abbreviations

ACTH	Adrenocorticotrophic hormone
ADH	Antidiuretic hormone
AFP	Alpha-fetoprotein
ALT	Alanine aminotransferase
ALL	Acute lymphoblastic leukaemia
AST	Aspartate aminotransferase
CEA	Carcinoembryonic antigen
CMV	Cytomegalovirus
DIC	Disseminated intravascular coagulation
HCG	Human chorionic gonadotrophin
5-HIAA	5-Hydroxyindole acetic acid
HVA	Homovanillic acid
MAO	Monoamine oxidase
MSH	Melanocyte stimulating hormone
PT	Prothrombin time
PTH	Parathyroid hormone
RT	Radiotherapy
PTT	Partial thromboplastin time
SIADH	Syndrome of inappropriate ADH secretion
VMA	Vanilmandelic acid

1 Introduction

1.1   Epidemiology

Cancer is the second most common cause of death in Great Britain after cardiovascular disease and there are approximately 10 000 cancer deaths in England and Wales each month. The 10 most common causes of death from cancer are shown in Table 1.1. It should be pointed out that where treatment has a significant effect on a tumour (e.g. testicular cancer or lymphoma) the prevalence of a disease will be much greater than indicated by mortality rates alone. Furthermore, such tumours will be much more commonly represented in a hospital population and have a proportionately greater amount of resources devoted to their care than the less responsive ones.

Over the past 50 years or so, substantial advances have taken place in the management of malignant disease. In the past, little could be done if surgery failed to eradicate a tumour but, advances in surgical technique, the development of safe, effective, radiotherapy and the advent of a large range of cytotoxic drugs and hormonal agents with activity against cancer mean that improvements in quality of life, and in some patients survival, is an attainable objective. The skill of a modern oncologist (surgical, radiological and

Table 1.1 Mortality from cancer (UK 1985)

	Mortality (numbers of deaths)		Rate per 100 000 pop.	
	Male	Female	Male	Female
Lung	29 543	11 317	1071	390
Breast	–	15 073	–	519
Prostate	7314	–	265	–
Stomach	6616	4596	240	158
Colon	5584	7168	203	247
Ovary	–	4290	–	148
Rectum	3659	3107	133	107
Cervix	–	2198	–	76
Pancreas	3410	3396	124	117
Bladder	3571	1608	130	55

1   Introduction

1.1   Epidemiology

medical) is in applying the right treatment at the right time and in knowing when it is best not to treat at all.

Estimates of the overall cure rate for cancer vary from 25 to 41% in developed countries and depend on how and where the analysis was made. The types of tumours included or excluded (e.g. skin

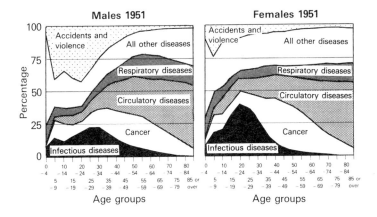

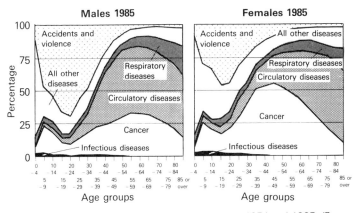

Fig. 1.1 Selected causes of death: by sex and age, 1951 and 1985. (From the Office of Population Censuses and Surveys, *Social Trends* **18**, 1988.)

1 Introduction

1.1 Epidemiology

tumours), the accuracy of the data collection services, the extent of underdiagnosis (especially in elderly patients) and, most important of all, the definition of cure employed, all affect the apparent 'cure' rate. The 5-year survival is the traditional indicator of curability and relies on the assumption that patients surviving for 5 years following the initial diagnosis are free of disease and unlikely to relapse subsequently. This will overestimate the incidence of 'cures', as some tumours continue to relapse up to 10 years or more after apparently successful treatment.

The incidence of cancer varies with age and is now a major cause of death in the UK population (Fig. 1.1). The incidence of, and deaths

Age-standardized mortality rates 1951 – 85 England and Wales

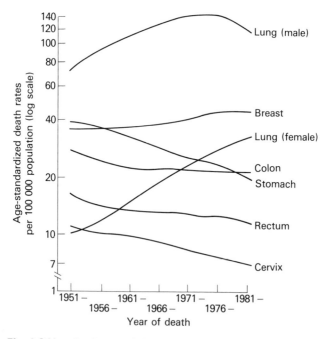

Fig. 1.2 Mortality time trends for common cancers in England and Wales

from, certain tumours are falling, while those of others are rising (Fig. 1.2), presumably because of environmental factors. This makes the true impact of modern cancer treatment all the more difficult to assess. For some tumours, however, there is strong evidence that advances in treatment over the last 10 years have produced quantifiable beneficial effects on a defined population.

New therapeutic approaches are continually being evaluated in clinical trials. The most rigorous test of a new treatment is the randomized controlled trial but many studies continue to be published using matched historical controls or natural history data banks. The latter are much easier to obtain and the ethical problems involved in the execution of such studies are less formidable, although the conclusions derived are harder to substantiate.

In spite of widespread public and, indeed often medical, pessimism, life today for the cancer patient is of better quality than it was in the past and often lasts longer. Perhaps more important, there is evidence of improvement in prognosis for patients with some tumours, which should give hope to those who suffer from what is still the most feared of all diseases.

1.2   Principles of cancer management

Cancer is the collective term for a group of over 200 diseases, which have in common a growth-regulatory defect which enables the tumours to invade tissue locally and to disseminate throughout the body. It is not the intention of this book to describe the management of these individual tumours but there are certain fundamental principles that are essential to the good management of patients with cancer.

Diagnosis

It is important to confirm the diagnosis by histology or cytology (see section 2.2), not only to be sure that the patient does have a malignant tumour but also because precise histology may influence the choice of treatment and give a guide to prognosis. There are occasional situations where it is obvious that a patient has cancer,

5

when biopsy may be difficult or hazardous and the result unlikely to influence treatment. These should, however, be uncommon exceptions to the rule.

Extent of disease

An attempt should be made to define the extent of disease or 'stage' the patient (see section 2.1). This should be based initially on clinical examination, blood tests and simple X-rays. In some situations, more invasive investigations, including laparotomy, may be justified but only if the results will influence the patient's eventual treatment.

Performance status

An assessment should be made of the patient's performance status or general fitness (see section 2.4), because this may reflect prognosis and influence the choice of treatment.

Treatment

When the basic information on diagnosis, stage and performance status is available, a clear decision should then be made as to whether to attempt to cure or palliate the patient's disease or to give symptomatic treatment alone.

Curative

Curative treatment is an attempt to destroy all malignant cells with one particular treatment or a combination of different ones. Such treatment must not only be directed at the primary tumour but also at all possible sites of local invasion or metastasis. For most solid tumours that are apparently localized, surgical excision is the treatment of choice and this may be followed by radiotherapy to the site of excision and/or adjuvant chemotherapy (see below). Curative treatment with radiotherapy (see section 3.4) is used when a localized tumour is surgically inoperable or when defined local spread may have occurred but disseminated metastases are unlikely (e.g. early carcinoma of the cervix or Hodgkin's disease). When the tumour is widely disseminated (e.g. leukaemia or a solid tumour with multiple metastases), chemotherapy is the only method of attempting curative treatment (although it may be combined with radiotherapy and/or surgery). Chemotherapy is only likely to result in long-term cures in a few very responsive tumours (e.g. the lymphomas, teratoma, childhood leukaemia) but applying the principles of curative treatment may prolong survival even if relapse eventually occurs.

Palliative

Palliative treatment is an attempt to relieve symptoms caused by a tumour, using specific antitumour therapy, with no intention and little expectation of cure. The symptoms should be carefully evaluated before and at regular intervals during, treatment and if there is no obvious response or unacceptable toxicity, treatment should be discontinued. Palliative chemotherapy should be given for at least 2 courses or 2 months, unless obvious progression occurs, if it is to have an adequate trial.

Symptomatic

Symptomatic treatment is the relief of symptoms using therapy with no direct antitumour effect. The most obvious example of this is the use of analgesics.

Adjuvant therapy

This is a term applied to chemotherapy or hormone therapy given after local treatment, in tumours where dissemination is undetectable but can be assumed to have occurred. If effective, it should lead to a significant increase in the cure rate or overall disease-free survival. A theoretical advantage of adjuvant therapy is that treatment is given when the tumour volume is very small and apparently more sensitive to anticancer drugs. A number of points should be made about adjuvant therapy:

- its value has not yet been convincingly proved in any tumour

although a case for its use is accumulating for breast cancer
- long-term side-effects, such as sterility and secondary malignancy assume greater importance for younger patients or where prolonged survival can be anticipated (see section 5.3).
- morbidity and mortality from the short-term side-effects should ideally be low
- it can, at present, be recommended only in the context of clinical trials

Response
At the end of any course of treatment, an attempt should be made to assess the response (see section 2.5), by noting any change in performance status, symptoms and objective measurements of the tumour. This may necessitate repeating some or all of the initial staging investigations which were originally abnormal. The assessment of response should be clearly recorded before proceeding to further therapy.

Follow-up
Patients should be followed up regularly after treatment and follow-up continued indefinitely (though at increasingly longer intervals), even in patients remaining apparently disease-free. This is not only because of the risk of late relapse in some tumours (especially breast carcinoma and Hodgkin's disease) but, also, to check for any long-term toxicity (see section 5.3) and to record the patient's overall survival (see section 2.5).

Patient confidence
Cancer is a frightening disease for patients and the treatment is often complex and toxic. It is, therefore, very important to gain the patient's confidence and to allow time to explain everything clearly and answer questions as honestly and as fully as possible. This is particularly so at the start of treatment and whenever treatment is stopped or changed. Equally, it is essential to make sure that the patient's family practitioner is kept fully informed of diagnosis,

prognosis, treatment and toxicity and also of what the patient has been told about his or her illness.

Terminology

The following terms are often used to describe the phases of chemotherapy and need definition.

Induction (or remission induction) treatment is the initial phase of intensive chemotherapy when an attempt is made to induce a complete remission (see section 2.5).

Consolidation treatment is chemotherapy given after achieving complete remission (in particular for acute leukaemia), in an attempt to make such a remission durable. It usually consists of the same intensive chemotherapy as remission induction, repeated for a limited number of courses.

Maintenance treatment is given to maintain complete remission. It is usually less intensive and given less frequently but carried on for a prolonged period, perhaps up to 2 years. It would only be used in conditions where its role is well established.

Late intensification describes intensive chemotherapy, perhaps the same as used during the initial induction phase, given at the end of a prolonged period of complete remission and maintenance treatment.

Cranial prophylaxis is the use of cranial or craniospinal irradiation or intrathecal chemotherapy either alone or in combination when complete remission has been achieved in tumours where there is a high likelihood of relapse within the central nervous system, e.g. lymphoblastic leukaemia and some lymphomas.

2   Assessment

2.1   Staging classifications

Staging is a measure of the extent of tumour in a particular patient. Its purpose is to categorize the wide range of clinical presentations into groups with common prognoses and patterns of disease in order to help select a suitable treatment policy. The principal treatment decision to be made is whether local, systemic or combined modality treatment is most appropriate. Staging can also be used to define accurately the extent of disease for trial stratification and, frequently, correlates well with prognosis. Staging may be either 'clinical' (essentially non-invasive) — based on physical examination, together with biochemical, immunological and imaging techniques — or pathological — based on histologically proven sites of disease. The latter is much more rigorous but where the result of an invasive staging procedure will not alter treatment outcome or management of a patient, it is not justified to subject that patient to the morbidity of the investigation. The financial cost of staging procedures can also be high and may be a major factor where resources are limited.

For most tumours, there is a simple system for classifying the extent of disease into 3 or 4 stages, which has practical use in deciding treatment and predicting prognosis. More complex and detailed classifications have been devised for many tumours, based on the tumour, nodes, metastases (TNM) system and depending often on accurate surgical and pathological information. For some tumours (e.g. breast and bladder carcinomas), TNM staging has therapeutic and prognostic importance, though this is generally restricted to surgical treatments. As well as the complexity of many staging systems there is a further problem caused by the number of systems available for any one tumour.

Internationally agreed staging systems are useful for comparing results between centres but suffer from the drawback that they depend on how carefully staging investigations are done. The more sensitive the method of assessment, the more likely it is that a patient will be categorized as having an advanced stage which, in turn, may alter the treatment and affect trial analysis. Because of

2.1   Staging classifications

improving staging investigations there is a tendency with time for patients with less advanced disease to be placed in each staging group. This process is known as stage migration or the Will Rogers phenomenon and means that it is not valid to compare the results, stage for stage, of trials that have used staging procedures of different sensitivity.

Many staging systems use the TNM system. Full details on the commonest staging systems can be found in: *TNM Classification of Malignant Tumours* (4th edition), UICC, Springer-Verlag 1987 or *Manual Staging of Cancer* (3rd edition), AJCC, JB Lippincott Co. 1988.

Breast carcinoma

The TNM classification of breast cancer (UICC 1987) is widely used and is shown here in full. A more recent introduction is stage grouping (Table 2.1). This complex staging system is summarized in Table 2.2.

Table 2.1. Stage grouping

Stage	Tumour	Nodes	Metastases
0	Tis	N0	M0
I	T1	N0	M0
II$_A$	T0	N1	M0
	T1	N1	M0
	T2	N0	M0
II$_B$	T2	N1	M0
	T3	N0	M0
III$_A$	T0	N2	M0
	T1	N2	M0
	T2	N2	M0
	T3	N2,N2	M0
III$_B$	T4	Any N	M0
	Any T	N3	M0
IV	Any T	Any N	M1

2 Assessment

2.1 Staging classifications

Table 2.2. Summary of the staging system for breast carcinoma

Tis	*In situ*
T1	≤2 cm
$T1_a$	≤0.5 cm
$T1_b$	>0.5 to 1 cm
$T1_c$	>1 to 2 cm
T2	>2 to 5 cm
T3	>5 cm
T4	Chest wall/skin
$T4_a$	Chest wall
$T4_b$	Skin oedema/ulceration, satellite skin nodules
$T4_c$	Both 4_a and 4_b
$T4_d$	Inflammatory carcinoma
N1	Movable axillary
	pN1
	pN1a Micrometastasis only ≤0.2 cm
	pN1b Gross metastasis
	i 1–3 nodes/>0.2 to <2 cm
	ii ≥4 nodes/>0.2 to <2 cm
	iii through capsule/<2 cm
	iv ≥2 cm
N2	Fixed axillary pN2
N3	Internal mammary pN3

Clinical

T — tumour

TX   Primary tumour cannot be assessed

T0   No evidence of primary tumour

Tis   Carcinoma *in situ:* intraductal carcinoma, or lobular carcinoma *in situ,* or Paget's disease of the nipple with no tumour

T1   Tumour 2 cm or less in greatest dimension

      $T1_a$ 0.5 cm or less in greatest dimension

      $T1_b$ More than 0.5 cm but not more than 1 cm in greatest dimension

      $T1_c$ More than 1 cm but not more than 2 cm in greatest dimension

2   Assessment

2.1   Staging classifications

T2   Tumour more than 2 cm but not more than 5 cm in greatest dimension

T3   Tumour more than 5 cm in greatest dimension

T4   Tumour of any size with direct extension to chest wall or skin

   $T4_a$ Extension to chest wall

   $T4_b$ Oedema (including peau d'orange), or ulceration of the skin of the breast, or satellite skin nodules confined to the same breast

   $T4_c$ Both 4_a and 4_b above

   $T4_d$ Inflammatory carcinoma

N — regional lymph nodes

NX   Regional lymph nodes cannot be assessed (e.g. previously removed)

N0   No regional lymph node metastasis

N1   Metastasis to movable ipsilateral axillary node(s)

N2   Metastasis to ipsilateral axillary node(s) fixed to one another or to other structures.

N3   Metastasis to ipsilateral internal mammary lymph node(s)

M — distant metastasis

MX   Presence of distant metastasis cannot be assessed

M0   No distant metastasis

M1   Distant metastasis (includes metastasis to supraclavicular lymph nodes)

Pathological

pT — primary tumour

The pathological classification requires the examination of the primary carcinoma with no gross tumour at the margins of resection. A case can be classified pT if there is only microscopic tumour in a margin.

   The pT categories correspond to the T categories.

2.1   Staging classifications

pN — regional lymph nodes

The pathological classification required the resection and examination of at least 6 or more lymph nodes.

pNX   Regional lymph nodes cannot be assessed (not removed for study or previously removed)

pN0   No regional lymph node metastasis

pN1   Metastasis to movable ipsilateral axillary node(s)

    pN1$_a$ Only micrometastasis (not larger than 0.2 cm)

    pN1$_b$ Metastasis to lymph node(s), any larger than 0.2 cm

        pN1$_{bi}$ Metastasis in 1–3 lymph nodes, any more than 0–2 cm and all less than 2.0 cm in greatest dimension

        pN1$_{bii}$ Metastasis to 4 or more lymph nodes, any more than 0.2 cm and all less than 2.0 cm in greatest dimension

        pN1$_{biii}$ Extension of tumour beyond the capsule of a lymph node metastasis less than 2.0 cm in greatest dimension

        pN1$_{biv}$ Metastasis to a lymph node 2.0 cm or more in greatest dimension

pN2   Metastasis to ipsilateral axillary lymph nodes that are fixed to one another or to other structures

pN3   Metastasis to ipsilateral internal mammary lymph node(s)

pM—distant metastasis

The pM categories correspond to the M categories.

Chronic lymphocytic leukaemia (Rai *et al.,* 1975)

Stage 0 patients are diagnosed by chance. The degree of lymphocytosis in stage 0 is arbitrary but excludes reactive lymphocytosis, while maintaining the overlap with some forms of malignant lymphoma. The rate of progression is also an important prognostic feature.

0   Lymphocytosis ($>15 \times 10^9$/l)

    Lymphocytes $>40\%$ of nucleated cells in bone marrow

2.1   Staging classifications

I   As 0 but with enlarged lymph nodes
II   As 0 but with enlarged spleen or liver or both; nodes may or
      may not be enlarged
III   As 0, I or II but Hb concentration <11 g/dl
IV   As 0, II or III but platelet count $<100 \times 10^9$/dl

Bladder carcinoma

UICC TNM clinical classification (1987)

T — primary tumour
The suffix 'm' should be added to the appropriated T category to
indicate multiple tumours. The suffix 'is' may be added to any 'T' to
indicate presence of associated carcinoma *in situ.*

TX   Primary tumour cannot be assessed
T0   No evidence of primary tumour
Tis   Carcinoma *in situ*: 'flat tumour'
T_a Non-invasive papillary carcinoma
T1   Tumour invades subepithelial connective tissue
T2   Tumour invades superficial muscle (inner half)
T3   Tumour invades deep muscle or perivesical fat
       $T3_a$ Tumour invades deep muscle (outer half)
       $T3_b$ Tumour invades perivesical fat
T4   Tumour invades any of the following: prostate, uterus,
       vagina, pelvic wall, abdominal wall

Note: If pathology report does not specify that tumour invades
muscle, consider as invasion of subepithelial connective tissue. If
depth of muscle invasion is not specified by the surgeon, code as
T2.

pTNM pathological classification
The pT, pN and pM categories correspond to the T, N and M
categories.
$T3_b$ Invasion through the full thickness of bladder wall

2.1   Staging classifications

T4   Tumour fixed or invading neighbouring structures and/or there is microscopic evidence of invasion of the prostate and in the other circumstances listed below at least muscle invasion

$T4_a$ Tumour invading substance of prostate, uterus, or vagina

$T4_b$ Tumour fixed to the pelvic wall and/or infiltrating the abdominal wall

Nodal involvement (N)

The regional lymph nodes are pelvic nodes just below the bifurcation of the common iliac arteries. The juxtaregional lymph nodes are the inguinal nodes, the common iliac, and para-aortic nodes.

NX   Minimum requirements cannot be met

N0   No involvement of regional lymph nodes

N1   Involvement of a single homolateral regional lymph node

N2   Involvement of contralateral, bilateral or multiple regional lymph nodes

N3   There is a fixed mass on the pelvic wall with a free space between this and the tumour

N4   Involvement of juxtaregional lymph nodes

Distant metastasis (M)

MX   Not assessed

M0   No (known) distant metastasis

M1   Distant metastasis present

American Joint Committee TNM classification (1978)

Primary tumour (T)

The suffix 'm' should be added to the appropriate T category to indicate multiple lesions. Papilloma is classified as 'G0'.

TX   Minimum requirements cannot be met

T0   No evidence of primary tumour

Tis   Sessile carcinoma *in situ*

T_a Papillary non-invasive carcinoma

2 Assessment

2.1 Staging classifications

T1 On bimanual examination a freely mobile mass may be felt; this should not be felt after complete transurethral resection of the lesion and/or there is papillary carcinoma without microscopic invasion beyond the lamina propria

T2 On bimanual examination there is induration of the bladder wall, which is mobile. There is no residual induration after complete transurethral resection of the lesion and/or there is microscopic invasion of superficial muscle of bladder

T3 On bimanual examination there is induration or a nodular mobile mass is palpable in the bladder wall which persists after transurethral resection

    $T3_a$ Microscopic invasion of deep muscle

    $T3_b$ Tumour with invasion of perivesical fissure

UICC stage grouping

Stage 0	Tis	N0	M0
	T_a	N0	M0
Stage I	T1	N0	M0
Stage II	T2	N0	M0
Stage III	$T3_a$	N0	M0
	$T3_b$	N0	M0
Stage IV	T4	N0	M0
	Any T	N1, N2, N3	M0
	Any T	Any N	M1

Carcinoma of the cervix uteri

TNM clinical and pathological classification

Comparison of UICC (1987) and FIGO systems

TNM categories	FIGO stages	
TX	–	Primary tumour cannot be assessed
T0	–	No evidence of primary tumour

2 Assessment

2.1 Staging classifications

TNM	FIGO	
Tis	0	Carcinoma *in situ*
T1	I	Cervical carcinoma confined to uterus (extension to corpus should be disregarded)
T1$_a$	I$_a$	Preclinical invasion carcinoma, diagnosed by microscopy only
T1$_{a1}$	I$_{a1}$	Minimal microscopic stromal invasion
T1$_{a2}$	I$_{a2}$	Tumour with invasive component 5 mm or less in depth taken from the base of the epithelium, and 7 mm or less in horizontal spread
T1$_b$	I$_b$	Tumour larger than T1$_{a2}$
T2	II	Cervical carcinoma invades beyond uterus but not to pelvic wall or to lower third of the vagina
T2$_a$	II$_a$	Without parametrial invasion
T2$_b$	II$_b$	With parametrial invasion
T3	III	Cervical carcinoma extends to pelvic wall and/or involves the lower third of the vagina and/or causes hydronephrosis or non-functioning kidney
T3$_a$	III$_a$	Tumour involves lower third of the vagina, no extension to pelvic wall
T3$_b$	III$_b$	Tumour extends to pelvic wall and/or causes hydronephrosis or non-functioning kidney
T4	IV$_a$	Tumour invades mucosa of bladder or rectum and/or extends beyond true pelvis *Note:* the presence of bullous oedema is not sufficient evidence to classify a tumour T3
M1	IV$_b$	Distant metastasis

2   Assessment

2.1   Staging classifications

N — regional lymph nodes
NX   Regional lymph nodes cannot be assessed
N0   No regional lymph node metastasis
N1   Regional lymph node metastasis

M — distant metastasis
MX   Presence of distant metastasis cannot be assessed
M0   No distant metastasis
N1   Distant metastasis

Colonic carcinoma
Various modifications have been proposed to the original Duke's classification shown below. These have subdivided the B category by depth of invasion and the C group by number of lymph nodes positive.

Duke's classification
A   Confined to the mucosa and submucosa
B   Spread through the muscularis
C   Spread to local lymph nodes
D   Distant metastasis present

UICC TNM clinical and pathological classification (1987)

T — primary tumour
TX   Primary tumour cannot be assessed
T0   No evidence of primary tumour
Tis   Carcinoma *in situ*
T1   Tumour invades submucosa
T2   Tumour invades muscularis propria
T3   Tumour invades through muscularis propria into subserosa or into non-peritonealized pericolic or perirectal tissues
T4   Tumour perforates the visceral peritoneum or directly invades other organs or structures

2   Assessment

2.1   Staging classifications

N — regional lymph nodes

NX   Regional lymph nodes cannot be assessed
N0   No regional lymph node metastasis
N1   Metastasis in 1 to 3 pericolic or perirectal lymph nodes
N2   Metastasis in 4 or more pericolic or perirectal lymph nodes
N3   Metastasis in any lymph node along the course of a named vascular trunk

M — distant metastasis

MX   Presence of distant metastasis cannot be assessed
M0   No distant metastasis
M1   Distant metastasis

Stage grouping for colon and rectum

	Tumour	Nodes	Metastasis	Duke's
Stage 0	Tis	N0	M0	
Stage I	T1	N0	M0	A
	T2	N0	M0	
Stage II	T3	N0	M0	B1
	T4	N0	M0	
Stage III	Any T	N1	M0	C1
	Any T	N2, N3	M0	
Stage IV	Any T	Any N	M1	

Note: Duke's B is a composite of better (T3N0M0) and worse (T4N0M0) prognostic groups, as is Duke's C (any TN1M0 and any TN2, 3M0).

Head and neck tumours

It is impossible to include the various sites under one heading and the groups below should be used as a guide only. Reference should be made to the UICC manual on staging for the TNM classification.

2 Assessment

2.1 Staging classifications

I   T1 tumour without spread
II T2 tumour without spread
III Tumour with local infiltration (T3) and/or mobile ipsilateral nodes 3 cm or less in greatest dimension (N1)
IV Extension to bone, muscle, skin, antrum and/or fixed or mobile nodes

Hodgkin's disease and lymphomas (Ann Arbor classification)
The same classification is applied to both diseases, although in Hodgkin's disease spread is through contiguous node groups, usually from the neck through mediastinum, para-aortic nodes and spleen, whereas in lymphomas it is much less predictable and the Ann Arbor classification is not very meaningful for them. Laparotomy is widely performed in early Hodgkin's (I–III$_a$), which is the group for which local treatment is of value but it is not usually done in non-Hodgkin's lymphomas.

I   Single node group
II   Two or more node group same side of diaphragm
III   Node groups both sides of diaphragm
   III$_i$ Involvement limited to the splenic hilar and coeliac nodes
   III$_{ii}$ Involvement of para-aortic lymph nodes
   III$_s$ Spleen involvement
IV   Diffuse extranodal involvement

A   No symptoms
B   Weight loss (10%)/fever/sweating
E   Localized extranodal involvement
(Carbone *et al.*, 1971)

2.1   Staging classifications

Ovarian carcinoma

TNM clinical and pathological classification

Comparison of UICC (1987) and FIGO systems

TNM categories	FIGO stages	
TX		Primary tumour cannot be assessed
T0		No evidence of primary tumour
T1	I	Tumour limited to ovaries
$T1_a$	I_a	Tumour limited to 1 ovary; capsule intact, no tumour on ovarian surface
$T1_b$	I_b	Tumour limited to both ovaries; capsules intact, no tumour on ovarian surface
$T1_c$	I_c	Tumour limited to 1 or both ovaries with any of the following: capsule ruptured, tumour on ovarian surface, malignant cells in ascites or peritoneal washing.
T2	II	Tumour involves one or both ovaries with pelvic extension
$T2_a$	II_a	Extension and/or implants on uterus and/or tube(s)
$T2_b$	II_b	Extension to other pelvic tissues
$T2_c$	II_c	Pelvic extension (2_a or 2_b) with malignant cells in ascites or peritoneal washing
T3 and/or N1	III	Tumour involves one or both ovaries with microscopically confirmed peritoneal metastasis outside the pelvis and/or regional lymph node metastasis
$T3_a$	III_a	Microscopic peritoneal metastasis beyond pelvis
$T3_b$	III_b	Macroscopic peritoneal metastasis beyond pelvis 2 cm or less in greatest dimension

2.1   Staging classifications

T3$_c$ and/or N1 III$_c$		Peritoneal metastasis beyond pelvis more than 2 cm in greatest dimension and/or regional lymph node metastasis
M1	IV	Distant metastasis (excludes peritoneal metastasis)

Note: Liver capsule metastasis is T3/stage III, liver parenchymal metastasis M1/stage IV. Pleural effusion must have positive cytology for M1/stage IV.

Malignant melanoma

Although there is a UICC TNM system, prognosis in melanoma is best predicted by the measured depth of invasion, together with the site of the primary, the trunk being worse than the limbs. Clark's levels are shown for comparison. Grouping by extent of metastases has little value, in view of the poor response of this tumour to chemotherapy.

Clark's levels		Depth of invasion
I	Atypical melanocytic hyperplasia	<0.75 mm
II	Tumour involving papillary dermis	<0.75 mm
III	Tumour extending to but not invading reticular dermis	0.75–1.5 mm
IV	Tumour invading reticular dermis	1.4–2.99 mm
V	Tumour invading subcutaneous tissue	>3.00 mm

Myeloma (Durie and Salmon, 1975)

Stage 1. Low myeloma cell mass ($<0.6 \times 10^{12}$ cells/m^2)
   Criteria
   All of the following:
   Hb >10 g/dl
   Serum Ca^{2+} <3.0 mmol/l
   X-rays: normal bone structure or solitary lesion only
   M-component production rates:
      IgG <50 g/l

2.1   Staging classifications

IgA <30 g/l
Urine light chain excretion <4 g/24 h

Stage II. Intermediate myeloma cell mass ($0.6-1.2 \times 10^{12}$ cells/m^2)
   Criteria
   Fitting neither stage I nor III

Stage III. High myeloma cell mass ($>1.2 \times 10^{12}$ cell/m^2)
   Criteria
   Any of the following:
   Hb <8.5 g/dl
   Serum Ca^{2+} >3.0 mmol/l
   Advanced lytic bone lesions
   M-component production rates:
      IgG value > 70 g/l
      IgA value >50 g/l
      Urine light chain excretion >4 g/24 h

Subclassified A or B, according to the absence or presence of renal
impairment, respectively.

Lung carcinoma

Non-small cell
(UICC TNM clinical and pathological classification, 1987)

T — primary tumour
TX   Primary tumour cannot be assessed, or tumour proven by
      the presence of malignant cells in sputum or bronchial
      washings but not visualized by imaging or bronchoscopy
T0   No evidence of primary tumour
Tis   Carcinoma *in situ*
T1   Tumour 3 cm or less in greatest dimension, surrounded by
      lung or visceral pleura, without bronchoscopic evidence of
      invasion more proximal than the lobar bronchus (i.e. not in
      the main bronchus)

2 Assessment

2.1 Staging classifications

T2   Tumour with any of the following features of size or extent:
More than 3 cm in greatest dimension
Involves main bronchus, 2 cm or more distal to the carina
Invades visceral pleura
Associated with atelectasis or obstructive pneumonitis which extends to the hilar region but does not involve the entire lung

T3   Tumour of any size which directly invades any of the following: chest wall (including superior sulcus tumours), diaphragm, mediastinal pleura, parietal pericardium; or tumour in the main bronchus less than 2 cm distal to the carina but without involvement of the carina; or associated atelectasis or obstructive pneumonitis of the entire lung

T4   Tumour of any size which invades any of the following: mediastinum, heart, great vessels, trachea, oesophagus, vertebral body, carina; or tumour with malignant pleural effusion

N — regional lymph nodes
NX   Regional lymph nodes cannot be assessed
N0   No regional lymph node metastasis
N1   Metastasis in ipsilateral peribronchial and/or ipsilateral hilar lymph nodes, including direct extension
N2   Metastasis in ipsilateral mediastinal and/or subcarinal lymph node(s)
N3   Metastasis in contralateral mediastinal, contralateral hilar, ipsilateral or contralateral scalene or supraclavicular lymph node(s)

M — distant metastasis
MX   Presence of distant metastasis cannot be assessed
M0   No distant metastasis
M1   Distant metastasis

2   Assessment

2.1   Staging classifications

Small cell lung cancer

This is a rapidly growing tumour which has frequently metastasized at the time of presentation; because of this the above TNM system is not very useful. The following simple classification is of greater practical and prognostic value:

Limited disease   Tumour confined to one hemithorax. Includes ipsilateral supraclavicular nodes but not where a pleural effusion is present

Extensive disease Spread beyond the limits described above

Testicular tumours

There are a number of staging system in addition to that quoted below.

Royal Marsden classification

I	Lymphogram negative, no evidence of metastasis
II	Lymphogram positive, metastases confined to abdominal nodes, 3 subgroups recognized
II_a	Maximum diameter of metastasis <2 cm
II_b	Maximum diameter of metastasis 2–5 cm
II_c	Maximum diameter of metastasis >5 cm
III	Involvement of supradiaphragmatic and infradiaphragmatic lymph nodes, no extralymphatic metastasis
IV	Extralymphatic metastasis. Suffixes: 0, lymphogram negative; a, b, and c, as for stage II

Lung status

L1	<3 metastases
L2	multiple <2 cm maximum diameter
L3	multiple >2 cm diameter

Liver status

H+   liver involvement

(Peckham *et al.*, 1979)

2 Assessment

2.1 Staging classifications

Uterine carcinoma (TNM clinical and pathological classification)

Comparison of UICC (1987) and FIGO classification

T — primary tumour

TNM categories	FIGO stages	
TX		Primary tumour cannot be assessed
T0		No evidence of primary tumour
Tis	0	Carcinoma *in situ*
T1	I	Tumour confined to corpus
T1$_a$	I$_a$	Uterine cavity 8 cm or less in length
T1$_b$	I$_b$	Uterine cavity more than 8 cm in length
T2	II	Tumour invades cervix but does not extend beyond uterus
T3	III	Tumour extends beyond uterus but not outside true pelvis
T4	IV$_a$	Tumour invades mucosa of bladder or rectum and/or extends beyond the true pelvis. *Note:* The presence of bullous oedema is not sufficient evidence to classify a tumour T4
M1	IV$_b$	Distant metastasis

Note: FIGO stages are further subdivided by histological grade:
G1   Well differentiated
G2   Moderately differentiated
G3–4 Poorly differentiated/undifferentiated

N — regional lymph nodes
NX   Regional lymph nodes cannot be assessed

2 Assessment

2.1 Staging classifications

N0   No regional lymph node metastasis
N1   Regional lymph node metastasis

M — distant metastasis
MX   Presence of distant metastasis cannot be assessed
M0   No distant metastasis
M1   Distant metastasis

2.2 Pathology

The aims of histopathology are:
- to give where possible a clear cut diagnosis
- histological grade or subtype
- extent of invasion (invasion of blood vessels, lymphatics, etc.)
- involvement of associated lymph nodes
- adequacy of the resection margins

Accurate histological diagnosis is essential at an early stage in management. This requires an adequate tissue sample, although treatment can be based on a needle biopsy or cytology, if this is diagnostic. Ideally, the results should always be discussed with the reporting pathologist as additional clinical information may help and the sureness of the diagnosis can be correctly gauged. Where there is doubt further studies or more tissue may be required or expert opinion sought.

Other tests which can contribute to the diagnosis and subtyping in some cases include:

1 Pre- and post-operative alpha-fetoprotein (AFP) and human chorionic gonadotrophin (HCG) may help in the diagnosis of testicular tumours (see section 2.3).

2 Urinary vanilmandelic acid (VMA) in suspected neuroblastomas and 5-hydroxyindole acetic acid (5-HIAA) in carcinoid tumours (see section 2.3).

3 Immunological studies.

4 Chromosomal studies are useful in the leukaemias and lymphomas.

5 Special stains and, more recently, immunocytochemistry and gene rearrangement studies often provide useful information in haematological malignancy but may cause a delay in diagnosis. Unfixed tissue is required for some of these tests.

6   Oestrogen and progesterone receptors are useful in selecting the best management of patients with breast cancer; these require unfixed tissue.

Whenever a biopsy is needed it is important that care should be taken so that the maximum information is obtained. The biopsy should be non-traumatized and fixed in small quantities, while keeping separate any samples required for frozen section or electron microscopy. Always check if unfixed tissue is required if a lymphoma is suspected.

2.3   Tumour markers

Biological markers of cancer may be derived from several sources:
- oncofetal antigens
- ectopic hormones
- enzymes
- products of tumour metabolism
- monoclonal antibodies

Though tumour markers are being actively sought and extravagant claims have been made for their use, they can only be used to optimize treatment and will make no impact on survival, unless effective therapy is available. They are useful in the following ways:
- To help establish the diagnosis of a particular tumour, e.g. the finding of a raised VMA helps confirm the diagnosis of neuroblastoma
- to monitor response to therapy, e.g. β-HCG and AFP in teratomas
- to monitor for early relapse after a complete remission
- as a potential tool in the screening for cancer
- for the localization of tumours by selective venous catheterization

The greatest problem in finding a useful tumour marker is the lack of specificity of most of the potential markers. Because of this, only a small number of markers are used clinically:
- alpha-fetoprotein (AFP)

2.3   Tumour markers

- carcinoembryonic antigen (CEA)
- β-human chorionic gonadotrophin (β-HCG)
- alkaline phosphatase
- acid phosphatase
- vanilmandelic acid (VMA)
- immunoglobulin production in multiple myeloma and some lymphomas
- 5-hydroxyindole acetic acid (5-HIAA)
- Ca 125 in ovarian carcinoma
- Placental alkaline phosphatase in seminoma
- Prostatic acid phosphatase in prostatic cancer
- β-2-microglobulin in myeloma

General principles for use
1   Always consider if there are other causes of a raised marker, apart from tumour.
2   If a tumour that commonly produces tumour markers is suspected, blood for levels of the appropriate markers should be taken prior to surgery. This particularly applies to any suspected teratoma.
3   After any treatment (surgical, radiotherapy or chemotherapy) in a patient with raised markers, serial blood tests for tumour markers should be taken to assess the response to that treatment. For some markers whose half-life is known (e.g. AFP and β-HCG), it is possible to plot the expected fall of the marker, assuming that treatment has destroyed or removed all the tumour producing the marker (e.g. surgical removal of a testicular teratoma). Comparison of the actual rate of fall of the blood markers with the expected fall will show if there is any remaining active tumour producing the marker. During prolonged treatment, such as chemotherapy, serial markers are obtained to ensure that the tumour is continuing to respond and the markers are falling.
4   After a complete remission (all tests normal including markers), follow-up marker studies can be used to detect relapse at an early stage.

2.3   Tumour markers

Alpha-fetoprotein (AFP)
This is a serum protein which is present at high concentration, prenatally. It is raised in malignant teratomas and in hepatocellular carcinoma. The half-life of AFP is 6 days. In the case of testicular tumours the presence of an elevated AFP almost certainly indicates the presence of teratomatous elements even if the histology is of a pure seminoma.

Non-malignant causes of a raised AFP include:
- viral hepatitis
- liver injuries causing hepatic regeneration
- inflammatory bowel disease
- during pregnancy (maternal and fetal blood)

Metastatic tumours in the liver, gall bladder carcinoma, prostatic carcinoma and lung cancer, are occasionally associated with a raised AFP.

β-human chorionic gonadotrophin (β-HCG)
With the introduction of radioimmunoassays, it has become possible to detect minute quantities of β-HCG. It is raised in choriocarcinomas and many teratomas. The half-life of β-HCG is about 30 hours. Moderate elevations of β-HCG are permissible in pure seminoma.

β-HCG is raised in a number of non-malignant conditions:
- pregnancy
- testicular failure in men (there may be some cross-reaction of luteinizing hormone (LH) with HCG in the assay)
- smokers of marijuana

β-HCG may also be raised in the presence of other tumours (liver, breast, stomach, pancreas and ovary).

Carcinoembryonic antigen (CEA)
The hopes for CEA as a tumour marker have not been fulfilled, mainly because of its lack of specificity. It is an oncofetal antigen and, in adults, was initially found in colon carcinoma, but it is also found in some patients with other tumours (breast, lung, pancreas, etc.).

2.3   Tumour markers
___

CEA is found in a wide variety of non-malignant conditions, including:
- heavy smokers
- inflammatory bowel diseases
- hepatitis
- cirrhosis
- pancreatitis
- recent blood transfusion
- gastritis

The major roles of CEA are to monitor response to therapy in colon and breast cancer, as a prognostic factor in colon cancer (raised levels at diagnosis indicate a worse outlook) and to detect early relapse. It is much less useful than β-HCG and AFP, partly because of its lack of specificity but, more importantly, because of the absence of effective treatments in the tumours in which it is found.

Alkaline phosphatase and placental alkaline phosphatase
Alkaline phosphatase derived from bone and liver, as well as ectopically synthesized placental alkaline phosphatase, can be used in the staging and monitoring of tumour response to therapy but, because elevation is very non-specific, its use is limited.

Prostatic acid phosphatase
This is raised in prostatic carcinoma and it is useful in diagnosis and monitoring of therapy. False-positives will result from haemolysis of blood samples.

Ca 125
This is a monoclonal antibody which interacts with determinants on about 80% of serous ovarian carcinomas. It's role as a marker is hampered by a lack of alternative therapy in the face of failure to respond or relapse.

Vanilmandelic acid (VMA)

VMA and homovanillic acid (HVA) are often elevated in neuroblastoma. They can be useful in making the diagnosis and for monitoring treatment. A major problem with this test is the need for a special diet (eliminating foods such as chocolate, bananas and vanilla). However if VMA, HVA, total metanephrines, cystathione and creatinine are measured in a 24-hour urine collection, no dietary restriction is needed, though drugs containing catecholamines should be avoided.

Immunoglobulins and Bence-Jones protein (light chains)

Myeloma cells and the malignant lymphocytes of some lymphomas may produce idiotypic antibodies. This is useful for confirming the diagnosis, by finding monoclonal immunoglobulin in the serum or urine (light chains) and by finding surface or intracellular monoclonal antibody, in malignant lymphoma cells.

The response of multiple myeloma can be followed by monitoring the serum immunoglobulins. Lymphomas rarely produce large quantities of immunoglobulins which can be monitored in plasma but the presence or absence of cells producing monoclonal antibodies may improve our ability to detect small numbers of malignant cells.

5-hydroxyindole acetic acid (5-HIAA)

Carcinoid tumours produce large amounts of 5-HIAA. The presence of increased amounts in the urine helps to confirm the diagnosis. Serial urinary 5-HIAA levels can also be used to monitor the response of the tumour to treatment.

Other tumour-secreting hormones

A number of tumours may produce hormones (some ectopically) which can be used to help make a diagnosis or to monitor response to therapy. These include:
- medullary carcinoma of the thyroid (parathyroid hormone [PTH])
- lung cancer, especially small cell (adrenocorticotrophic hormone

[ACTH], antidiuretic hormone [ADH], melanocyte-stimulating hormone [MSH], thyroid-stimulating hormone [TSH], etc.)
- pancreatic tumours (insulin, glucagon, gastrin)
- adrenal gland (ACTH, MSH)
- kidney (prolactin, PTH, renin, erythropoietin)
- rare ovarian tumours (17-ketosteroids)

2.4   Performance status

This arbitrary assessment of general well-being has been found to be remarkably useful in assessing prognosis and in the selection of patients suitable for intensive cytotoxic therapy. Many trials define a lower limit for inclusion in an attempt to limit morbidity and mortality attributable to non-malignant causes. Serial assessment by one observer also gives the most useful guide to progress and can be of help in making clinical decisions. Two scales are in common use and are described in Table 2.3. Undoubtedly, the correlation of performance status and results of cancer chemotherapy, depends on a number of interrelated factors such as age, stage, tumour bulk and extent of surgery if any, but in numerous studies it has emerged as an important prognostic variable, which is simple to use.

2.5   Response

Response is a measurable change in the size of a tumour. It is frequently used as a guide to prognosis and it provides a convenient end-point at which to take clinical decisions. The following 4 categories are commonly used:

1   Complete remission: disappearance of all recognizable tumour masses and/or biochemical changes directly related to the tumour and resolution of symptoms.

2   Partial remission: >50% decrease in all tumour masses, measured by the product of the longest $\times$ the widest perpendicular diameters.

3   Progressive disease: occurrence of any new lesion or increase in the longest $\times$ widest perpendicular diameters of measurable disease by more than a third.

2.5   Response

4   Stable disease: changes smaller than those described above.

Response indicates sensitivity to therapy but may not necessarily equate with survival. The minimum duration of remission usually accepted is 4 weeks but it should be remembered that the biological significance of this depends on the rate of growth of the tumour. Certainly, the duration of remission or disease-free survival is a much better index of the effect of treatment. Good data of this sort are difficult to obtain and few chemotherapy regimens have been assessed by the more rigorous criteria to date. Other end-points, such as increasing performance status or disease stabilization, may be just as important in some patients. Like staging, the value of response to the patient depends largely on the sensitivity of the methods used to measure disease. For instance, response in testicular teratomas is a relatively defined end-point because of the sensitive biochemical markers that are available and metastatic disease can generally be well seen on X-rays or on CT scans. By contrast, ovarian cancer, where spread is characterized by insidious intra-abdominal growth, is difficult to assess by current imaging techniques. 'Second-look' surgery cannot at present be recommended as a routine procedure in the absence of effective salvage therapy.

In general, there is only an increase in survival in patients who achieve a complete remission. A partial remission indicates significant drug activity and may be accompanied by a subjective improvement.

Survival, which is usually recorded as the time from diagnosis to death, is probably the best index of the efficacy of a particular treatment. But accurate survival data are often difficult to obtain (especially in tumours where there may be late relapses) and difficult to interpret, because allowance must be made for any subsequent treatment. This is particularly important where there is a very effective second-line treatment (e.g. chemotherapy for patients with Hodgkin's disease relapsing after radiotherapy).

Table 2.3. Two commonly used scales of performance status

Karnofsky scale		WHO performance scale (similar to ECOG)	
Scale	Performance	Scale	Performance
100	Normal, no complaints, no evidence of disease	0	Able to carry out all normal activity without restriction
90	Able to carry on normal activity, no special care is needed		
80	Normal activity with effort, some signs or symptoms of disease	1	Restricted in physically strenuous activity but ambulatory and able to carry out light work
70	Cares for self, unable to carry on normal activity or do active work		
60	Requires occasional assistance but is able to care for most of own needs	2	Ambulatory and capable of all self-care but unable to carry out any work; up and about more than 50% of waking hours
50	Requires considerable assistance and frequent medical care		

| 3 | Capable of only limited self-care; confined to bed or chair more than 50% of waking hours |
| 4 | Completely disabled; cannot carry on any self-care; totally confined to bed or chair |

Unable to care for self, requires equivalent of institutional or hospital care; disease may be progressing rapidly

40	Disabled, requires special care and assistance
30	Severely disabled, hospitalization is indicated, although death is not imminent
20	Very sick, hospitalization necessary, active supportive treatment necessary
10	Moribund, fatal processes progressing rapidly
0	Dead

2.6   Data collection

Chemotherapy records

It is essential that accurate details are recorded, preferably in duplicate, of all chemotherapy administered, e.g. in the patient's notes and on separate record cards or flow sheets. This applies to both oral and i.v. therapy and charts should incorporate an assess-

MEDICAL ONCOLOGY UNIT   Ht .1.9 m.. Wt .75 kg.

NAME: F. RANK. N. STEIN

HOSPITAL NO: 54321

			1 / 4 / 82		22 / 4 / 82	
			Hb: 13·3		HB: 12·0	
			WBC: 10·2		WBC: 4·8	
			Pls: 300		Pls: 250	
			WT: 75		WT: 75	
			SA: 2·0		SA: 2·0	

DRUG	Dose m²		COURSE NO.		COURSE NO.	
			Dose	Given	Dose	Given
CYCLOPHOSPHAMIDE	750 mg	IV	1500	✓	1500	✓
ADRIAMYCIN	50 mg	IV	100	✓	100	✓
VINCRISTINE	1·4 mg	IV	2	✓	2	✓
PREDNISOLONE	100 mg	O	200×	5	200×	5
	SIGNATURE		D. R. Acula		D. R. Acula	

TOXICITY

Karnofsky P.S.		7		8
Nausea & vomiting		0		2
Alopecia		0		1
Neuropathy		0		0
Mucositis		0		0
Cystitis		0		0

Fig. 2.1. Chemotherapy prescription sheet and assessment of toxicity.

2   Assessment

2.6   Data collection

ment of toxicity. A sample sheet where the toxicity is assessed on a modified WHO scale (Table 2.4) is shown in Fig. 2.1. The reason for a dose alteration or drug change should be clearly described, as it is almost impossible to assess retrospectively.

Surface area (SL) m² ..2.:.0......

13/5/82		/ /		/ /		/ /	
Hb: **12·0** WBC: **3·8** Pls: **200**		Hb: WBC: Pls:		Hb: WBC: Pls:		Hb: WBC: Pls:	
WT: **75** SA:		WT: SA:		WT: SA:		WT: SA:	
COURSE NO.		COURSE NO.		COURSE NO.		COURSE NO.	
Dose	Given	Dose	Given	Dose	Given	Dose	Given
1500	✓						
100	✓						
2	✓						
200	x 5						
D.R.ACULA							

10						
2						
2						
1						
1						
0						

2   Assessment

2.6   Data collection

Patient records

Doctors are notoriously bad at keeping records of patient data and the standard hospital case record is more orientated towards a diagnostic work-up than close monitoring of complex therapy. However, much can be achieved by organizing a simple system to collect and record some essential data. Exactly what information is recorded depends on the type of tumour, the availability of secretarial staff and whether the patient is part of a local or multicentre trial.

Frequent access to the patients' hospital notes is required to assess progress and check laboratory values. One advantage of laboratory values or X-rays is that the results are held on file at source and, if missing from the case notes, the information can be obtained retrospectively. Response is the most important clinical end-point to record because treatment is usually modified as a result. Simple clinical parameters that are an excellent guide to progress but often omitted are the patient's weight and performance status by one of the standard scales. Where a suitable marker is available, as in leukaemia (blast cell count), teratoma (AFP or β-HCG) and myeloma (immunoglobulin), it can be of great help in management to plot these on a chart showing the relationship to treatment cycles. Computerized sytems are being introduced in certain centres but their consideration is outside the scope of this book.

Table 2.4. Toxicity score

	0	1	2	3	4
Haemorrhage	None	Petechiae	Mild blood loss	Gross blood loss	Debilitating blood loss
Oral	None	Soreness/erythema	Erythema, ulcers, can eat solids	Ulcers, requires liquid diet only	Feeding not possible
Nausea/vomiting	None	Nausea	Transient vomiting	Vomiting, requiring therapy	Intractable vomiting
Diarrhoea	None	Transient <2 days	Tolerable but >2 days	Intolerable, requiring therapy	Haemorrhagic dehydration
Constipation*	None	Mild	Moderate	Abdominal distension	Distension and vomiting
Bilirubin	<20	20–39	40–84	85–169	> 170 μmol/l
AST	<50	50–99	100–199	200–399	> 400 μ/l
ALT	<45	45–89	90–179	180–359	> 360 μ/l
Alk. phos.	<340	340–699	700–1399	1400–2799	> 2800 μ/l
Urea	<8.0	8.0–15.9	16.0–31.9	32.0–63.9	>64 mmol/l
Serum creatinine	<150	150–299	300–399	600–1190	>1200 mmol/l
Proteinuria	None	1+, < 3 g/l	2–3+, 3–10 g/l	4+, >10 g/l	Nephrotic syndrome

Table 2.4. Toxicity score (contd)

	0	1	2	3	4
Cystitis	None	Mild frequency and dysuria	Severe frequency and dysuria	Frank haemorrhagic cystitis	Cystectomy needed
Sodium (low)	>130	129–120	119–110	109–100	<100 mmol/l
Calcium (low) (corrected for albumin)	>2.3	2.29–2.0	1.99–1.75	1.74–1.5	>1.5 mmol/l
Magnesium (low)	>7.0	0.69–0.60	0.59–0.40	0.39–0.20	<0.20 mmol/l
Pulmonary	None	Mild symptoms	Exertional dyspnoea	Dyspnoea at rest	Complete bed rest required
Fever-drug	None	Fever <38°C	Fever 38–40°C	Fever >40°C	Fever with hypotension
Allergic	None	Oedema	Bronchospasm, no parenteral therapy needed	Bronchospasm, parenteral therapy required	Anaphylaxis
Cutaneous	None	Erythema	Dry desquamation, vesiculation, pruritus	Moist desquamation	Exfoliative dermatitis necrosis requiring surgery
Rash	None	Mild (transient and/or localized)	Moderate (persistent and/or generalized)	Severe (confluent erythema)	Exfoliative dermatitis

Alopecia	None	Minimal hair loss	Moderate, patchy alopecia	Severe alopecia	Total alopecia
Infection (specify site)	None	Minor infection	Moderate infection	Major infection	Major infection with hypotension
Cardiac rhythm	Normal	Sinus tachycardia >110 at rest	Unifocal VE atrial arrhythmia	Multifocal VE	Ventricular tachycardia
Cardiac function	Normal	Asymptomatic, but abnormal cardiac sign	Transient symptomatic dysfunction, no therapy required	Symptomatic dysfunction, responsive to therapy	Symptomatic dysfunction, not responsive to therapy
Pericarditis	None	Asymptomatic effusion	Symptomatic, no tap required	Tamponade, tap required	Tamponade, surgery required
Raynaud's phenomenon	None	Occasional mild attacks	Frequent mild attacks	Frequent severe attacks	Gangrene
State of consciousness	Alert	Transient lethargy	Somnolent <50% of waking hours	Somnolent >50% of waking hours	Coma
Neuropathy	None	Paraesthesia and/or decreased tendon reflexes	Severe paraesthesia and/or mild weakness	Intolerable paraesthesia and/or marked motor loss	Paralysis

Table 2.4. Toxicity score (contd)

	0	1	2	3	4
Ototoxicity	None	Difficulty with faint speech, soft transient tinnitus	Frequent difficulty with faint speech, soft persistent tinnitus	Frequent difficulty with loud speech, loud tinnitus	Hears only shouted/amplified speech, if at all; severe tinnitus
Pain**	None	Mild	Moderate	Severe	Intractable

*Constipation does not include constipation resulting from narcotics. **Treatment-related pain, not disease-related pain.
ALT = Alanine aminotransferase. AST = Aspartate aminotransferase.
Alk. phos. = alkaline phosphatase.

3 Radiotherapy

3.1   General principles

Radiotherapy (RT) is the therapeutic use of high-energy ionizing radiations, either electromagnetic waves (X-rays and γ-rays) or subatomic particles (β-particles, high-energy electrons and neutrons). These radiations penetrate tissues to different depths according to their physical nature and energy, and deposit their energy in a series of physico-chemical reactions starting with an ionization (usually of a water molecule) and culminating in damage to DNA and so in the interference with cell division. This process is unselective and will occur in the cells of normal tissues as well as those of tumours. The therapeutic usefulness of RT therefore depends partly on the differential sensitivity of some tumours and partly on careful planning and dose prescription to minimize normal tissue damage.

3.2   Radiotherapy methods

External beam

This entails treating the relevant volume of the patient with radiation from a source mounted at some distance from the skin surface. This is the most frequently used method of RT and the most usual types of beam and their uses are listed in Table 3.1.

Advantages:
- versatility
- treatment of deep-seated tumours
- 'skin-sparing' effect of megavoltage beams
- outpatient treatment

Disadvantages:
- special staff to run and maintain machines
- high capital and maintenance costs
- irradiation of critical normal tissues may be dose-limiting
- systemic side-effects
- immobilization of patient
- treatment usually fractionated over several weeks

Table 3.1. External beam radiation types and uses

Radiation	Source	Energy	Typical uses
X-rays:			
Superficial	X-ray machine	60–150 keV	Radical treatment of superficial skin tumours
Orthovoltage	X-ray machine	250–300 keV	Palliative treatment of large skin or subcutaneous tumours, and bone metastases; some radical treatments, e.g. breast
Megavoltage	Linear accelerator	4–20 MeV	Radical and palliative treatment of deep-seated tumours
γ-rays	Cobalt-60	1.2 MeV	Radical treatment of especially head and neck and breast tumours; palliative treatment to many sites, e.g. bones, lymph nodes, brain
	Caesium-137	622 keV	Head and neck treatments; rarely used in UK
β-particles	Strontium-90	2.3 MeV	Mycosis fungoides and other very superficial skin conditions
High-energy electrons	Linear accelerator	2–20 MeV	Radical and palliative treatment of skin and superficial tumours

3.2   Radiotherapy methods

Brachytherapy

Brachytherapy involves the use of radioactive material emitting high-energy ionizing radiation made into *sealed sources,* either containers tubes or needles), wires or grains that be inserted directly into the tumour and adjacent normal tissues, or applied in a special holder to the surface of the tumour. The commonly used radioisotopes and their uses are listed in Table 3.2

There are three different methods:

Intracavitary

Special sealed sources are inserted into suitable body cavities, most usually uterus and vagina for treating carcinoma of cervix and endometrium. Under general anaesthetic, either the sources themselves can be inserted directly, or else flexible tubes are positioned through which the sources can be passed when the patient has returned to the ward, either manually or by using a remote 'after-loading' machine (e.g. Selectron). Each application may last for a few hours or up to a week, depending on the dose prescribed.

Interstitial

Radioactive sealed sources are inserted directly into the tumour and surrounding tissues. A variety of techniques are used, including:
- caesium-137 or radium-226 needles
- flexible iridium-192 wires passed through polythene tubes
- gold-198 grains injected with a special gun

Superficial

Some superficial skin tumours can be treated by constructing a close-fitting plastic mould containing appropriately distributed sealed sources, applied to the skin. This is then worn by the patient either continuously or intermittently (during waking hours) for an accurately prescribed time, usually 5–7 days.

Advantages:
- very high local dose to tumour
- small amount of normal tissue irradiated

3.2   Radiotherapy methods

Table 3.2. Commonly used radioisotopes for brachytherapy

Radioisotope	Half-life	Energy	Uses
Caesium-137	30 years	662 keV	Tubes for intracavitary use; needles for interstitial use
Radium-226	1620 years	1.1 MeV	Tubes and needles — now largely superseded by caesium-137
Gold-198	2.7 days	412 keV	Seeds for interstitial use and superficial moulds
Cobalt-60	5.3 years	1.2 MeV	Tubes for intracavitary use in Cathetron; plaques for uveal melanoma
Strontium-90	28 years	2.3 MeV	Plaques for superficial eye treatment
Iodine-131	8 days	360 keV 610 keV	Orally for thyroid tumours and thyrotoxicosis
Phosphorus-32	14.3 days	0.68 MeV	Orally or IV for polycythaemia rubra vera

- no systemic upset
- short overall treatment time
  Disadvantages:
- general anaesthetic (except for superficial)
- hospital admission
- local discomfort
- risk of staff exposure to radiation
- relatively few tumours suitable

Unsealed sources

Two radioisotopes are commonly used for oral or intravenous administration:

Iodine-131

Iodine-131 is given orally and taken up selectively in thyroid tissue and hormonally functional thyroid tumour tissue, resulting in localized irradiation. It is used to treat thyrotoxicosis, ablate residual thyroid tissue and treat functional thyroid carcinoma and metastases. Administration of doses greater than 555 MBq (15 mCi) entails admitting the patient and nursing in an approved isolated area.

Phosphorus-32

Phosphorus-32 is given orally or i.v. resulting in a 'whole body' dose of low-energy β-irradiation, and therefore bone marrow suppression. It is used mainly in treatment of polycythaemia rubra vera.

3.3   Radiation safety

Because of the known hazards, there are strict safety regulations controlling the therapeutic uses of radiation. It is beyond the scope of this book to describe these, but it is worth stressing that all staff involved in caring for patients undergoing radiotherapy, especially brachytherapy or from unsealed sources, should be monitored by wearing a film badge, be familiar with the regulations and local rules and know what to do in the event of a mishap and who the Radiation Safety Officer is.

3.4   Radiation dosage and fractionation

Dosage

The modern SI unit of radiotherapy 'absorbed dose' is the gray (Gy). The tissues have received 1 Gy when 1 joule of radiation energy is absorbed per kilogram.

The old unit, the rad, is equivalent to 0.01 Gy or 1 centigray (cGy). Although the gray is the internationally approved unit, many radiotherapy centres in the UK which have been used to expressing doses in rads now express them in centigrays.

The dose from a single field treatment is prescribed either at the skin surface as an 'applied' or 'incident' dose (a.d. or i.d.) or else at a given depth from the surface as a 'tumour dose (t.d.) at x cm'.

The dose from the frequently used 'parallel opposed pair' of treatment fields, when two identical fields are applied from opposite sides of the patient (resulting in a fairly uniform dose across the patient) is usually prescribed to the centre of the volume as a 'mid-plane' dose (m.p.d.).

When more complex planned treatments with multiple fields are used the intention is to produce a uniform dose distribution within the tumour volume or 'region of interest'. The distribution is never completely uniform and a 10% variation is usually considered acceptable. The dose is then prescribed as a 'tumour' dose. This may be the maximum dose in the volume, the minimum dose, or an average or 'modal' dose. Different departments may use different prescribing conventions and it is important to know which is used when comparing treatments.

Fractionation

In the early days of radiotherapy it was discovered empirically that a greater antitumour effect could be achieved for an equivalent amount of normal tissue (usually skin and mucosa) damage by 'fractionating' the dose, giving it in a series of daily treatments over a period of weeks.

A biological rationale for this technique has subsequently been established in laboratory experiments. In general the longer the total time and the greater the number of fractions, the higher is the dose that is needed to produce a given tumour effect and the less the risk of late normal tissue damage.

It is therefore important when discussing radiotherapy dosage to know not only the total dose, but also the time and the number of fractions.

Conventional fractionation is daily treatment, 5 days a week, with fractions of 200 cGy.

Hypofractionation is treating less often than daily (e.g. 2 or 3 times per week).

Hyperfractionation is treating more than once daily.

Accelerated fractionation is giving treatment daily but in fractions greater than 200 cGy, resulting in a shorter overall treatment time.

Radical treatment
A radical treatment involves treating the tumour and surrounding tissues that may be involved (e.g. adjacent lymph nodes) to the maximum tolerated dose. It is generally the tolerance of adjacent critical normal tissues that limits the dose that can be given and this is discussed below (see section 3.5).

Radical treatment will almost always produce some acute toxicity and a finite risk of severe long-term toxicity.

Palliative treatment
A palliative treatment involves prescribing a dose of radiation that is likely to relieve the patient's symptoms while causing minimal acute or long-term toxicity.

3.5   Toxicity of radiotherapy

Systemic toxicity
The incidence of systemic symptoms from RT is very variable. In general, the larger the fields treated, the larger the fractions and the more prolonged the treatment the greater the risk of patients encountering problems. Conversely, many patients having short courses of palliative treatment experience little systemic toxicity.

Tiredness and general malaise are the most common symptoms especially with large field treatments and patients may have to adapt their life-style accordingly during their treatment.

Nausea and anorexia occur particularly when the abdomen is irradiated, but can occur with other large field treatments.

Organ-specific toxicity
The commonest organ-specific toxicities of RT are listed in Tables 3.3 and 3.4.

Table 3.3 lists the acute toxicities that may be experienced during and within a few months of treatment. Again, there is considerable individual variation in susceptibility and the doses at which they occur are only an approximate guide. Management of the commoner of these problems is described in section 3.6.

Table 3.4 lists some of the long-term problems that may be caused by RT. Again, the doses are only an approximate guide and there are some patients, fortunately quite rare, whose tissues appear to be unusually sensitive and who may experience problems at lower doses.

The volume irradiated is important. Irradiation of a small part of the lung or liver or a short length of spinal cord may be of little consequence whereas the same dose applied to the whole organ or a great length of cord may be disastrous.

Most of these chronic problems probably result from obliterative arteritis due to RT damage to endothelial cells. The resulting

3.5   Toxicity of radiotherapy

Table 3.3 Acute toxicities of radiotherapy (RT) (dose in Gy, assuming conventional fractionation)

Organ	Toxicity	Dose (Gy)
Skin	Erythema	10–20
	Dry desquamation	40–50
	Moist desquamation (commonest in fair-skinned)	45–55
Mucous membranes	Mucositis	30–40
Cornea	Keratitis	40–50
GI tract	Nausea and vomiting	Any dose
	Diarrhoea	30–40
Bladder	Frequency and dysuria	40–50
Brain	Somnolence syndrome in children at 6 weeks after RT	10–20
Spinal cord	L'hermitte's syndrome	20–30
Lung	Pneumonitis, with cough, dyspnoea and CXR changes at 3–6 months after RT	35–50
Liver	Acute hepatitis	25–35
Bone marrow	Suppression especially of WCC and platelets, during wide field RT	10–20
Hair	Alopecia	30–40

CXR = chest X-ray.
WCC = white cell count.

Table 3.4 Chronic toxicities of radiotherapy (dose in Gy, assuming conventional fractionation)

Organ	Toxicity	Symptoms	Dose (Gy)
Skin	Telangiectasia	Cosmetic	50–60
	Fibrosis	Lump, scarring, deformity	50–60
	Necrosis	Ulceration	60
Salivary glands	Secretory failure	Dry mouth	30

3.5   Toxicity of radiotherapy

Lacrimal glands	Secretory failure	Dry eyes, kerato-conjuctivitis	30
Lacrimal duct	Fibrosis	Epiphora	50–60
Eye	Lens opacity	Usually asymptomatic	2
	Progressive cataract	Visual loss	8–10
	Retinal damage	Visual loss	50–60
Small bowel	Stricture	Intestinal obstruction	45–50
	Fistula	Diarrhoea, nutritional problems	45–50
Large bowel	Stricture	Intestinal obstruction	55–60
	Fistula	Diarrhoea	55–60
	Telangiectasia	Rectal bleeding	55–60
Kidney	Nephritis	Proteinurea, hypertension, renal failure	15–20
Ureter	Stricture	Obstructive uropathy	50–60
Bladder	Telangiectasia	Haematuria	50–60
	Fibrosis	Frequency, dysuria	50–60
Brain	Necrosis	CNS signs	55–60
Pituitary	Failure	Hypopituitarism	55–60
Spinal cord	Necrosis	Acute or progressive paraparesis	40–50
Brachial plexus	Fibrosis	Pain, dysaesthesia, weakness	55–60
Lung	Fibrosis	Cough, dyspnoea	40–50
Heart	Arteritis	Ischaemic changes	40–50
Liver	Fibrosis	Chronic hepatitis	30–50
Ovary	Failure	Amenorrhoea	5–20
Testis		Temporary azoospermia	0.5–1
		Permanent azoospermia	5–10
Lymphatics	Fibrosis	Lymphoedema	55–60
Bone	Epiphyseal damage	Growth disturbance	10
	Necrosis	Pain, fracture	60–65

symptoms are often similar to those caused by other intercurrent illnesses or by recurrent tumour and, before attributing a particular problem to the effects of RT, it is important to establish that the original RT was of a dose and distribution likely to cause it. Appropriate investigations should be undertaken with a biopsy if indicated, although there is a hazard of necrosis from biopsying RT-damaged tissues.

Chronic problems may be of more consequence in children because of greater sensitivity (often enhanced by the sensitizing effect of many chemotherapeutic agents) and the production of developmental abnormalities (especially growth disturbance if unfused epiphyses are irradiated).

3.6   Managing patients during radiotherapy

General care

Most patients are very apprehensive when they first attend for RT. It is therefore important to warn them of possible side-effects and to reassure them about those that they are unlikely to experience.

General tiredness and malaise is the most frequent side-effect of all but short palliative or superficial courses of RT. Patients should be advised to rest as much as possible during the weeks of treatment and warned that their energy level may not return to normal for several weeks or months after RT is finished.

Anorexia is quite common but only severe if the abdomen or pelvis are irradiated. Patients should be told to maintain a normal balanced diet as far as possible, and specific help and advice given to those with RT-induced oral or oesophageal mucositis (see later).

Skin care

Skin reactions are dose-related and so depend not only on the dose prescribed but also on the physical characteristics of the radiation and the RT technique used. Orthovoltage and electron beams deposit the maximum dose at the skin surface and so skin reactions are directly related to the applied dose; whereas megavoltage beams produce a degree of 'skin-sparing' because the maximum dose occurs at the 'build-up' depth below the skin surface (c. 0.5 cm for cobalt-60 and 1 cm for 5 MeV X-rays). This only applies, however, when the beam is more or less perpendicular to the skin. If it is tangential, less sparing occurs, which explains the greater reactions seen in areas like the axilla, perineum and natal cleft. Also, with higher energy megavoltage beams skin reactions can occur at the exit site of the beam, especially in thin patients.

Patients are usually advised not to wash the treated area during RT. This is partly so as not to erase any alignment marks and partly because severe reactions can be exacerbated if the skin gets very wet and macerated. However, with megavoltage treatments it should be possible for patients to wash occasionally provided they are gentle and do not soak, scrub or rub the treated area.

Patients should be given strict instructions not to apply any cosmetics, deodorants or proprietary ointments to the skin as they may exacerbate reactions (especially if they contain metals). Plain starch dusting powders can be used and may be soothing. Whenever feasible patients should wear loose-fitting clothes and avoid skin abrasion.

Erythema is common, occurring at a dose of about 10 Gy and may proceed to dry desquamation. Usually this requires no treatment but if severe and symptomatic the patient can be given either a simple emollient cream (e.g. E45) or 1% hydrocortisone cream (although there is no strong evidence that the corticosteroid is in fact helpful).

Moist desquamation is the most severe form of skin reaction and may necessitate suspension of RT to allow partial healing. It can usually be managed by keeping the affected area dry and free from abrasion by clothing. Crystal violet paint ('Gentian violet') is useful in drying the area and preventing secondary infection, although it is somewhat messy and unsightly.

Most patients who have had little or no skin reactions can resume washing as soon as RT is finished provided they are careful. But moist desquamation (especially if the skin received all of a radical dose) may take several weeks or months to heal, and patients may need regular care and help with dressings, etc. The main principle of treatment is to keep the area dry and clean to allow healing.

Mouth care
Dental and oral hygiene is very important for patients having radical RT to the head and neck. Whenever possible, dental treatment (including extractions) should be carried out before RT starts, as there is an increased risk of failure to heal and mandibular necrosis afterwards.

During treatment patients should maintain good oral hygiene with regular tooth-brushing and rinsing with dilute antiseptic and analgesic rinses and vigorous treatment of any secondary infection (see section 4.2). If it become severe and the patient is unable to eat or drink, RT may have to be suspended to allow some recovery, or fine-bore nasogastric feeding considered (see section 4.1).

Nausea and Vomiting
Some nausea and anorexia may occur during any but the most brief or superficial course of RT, but vomiting is unusual unless the upper abdomen is irradiated. It should be managed with simple anti-emetics (see section 4.2) given regularly. When a planned course of RT is very likely to produce severe nausea (e.g. para-aortic node irradiation for Hodgkin's disease or seminoma) it is worthwhile starting anti-emetics before the first treatment.

Dysphagia
Dysphagia due to oesophageal mucositis may occur during or after a course of thoracic RT. It can be helped by antacid and local anaesthetic suspension (Mucaine) or an alginate/antacid mixture if there is a history of reflux. Any hint of candidal superinfection should be investigated and treated appropriately (see section 4.3).

Diarrhoea
Diarrhoea is an inevitable complication of most abdominal and pelvic

RT treatments. It starts at a dose of 20–30 Gy and may persist for some weeks after the RT has finished. Patients at risk should be advised to take a low-residue diet and given conventional constipating agents (see section 4.2).

Bladder disturbance

Frequency and dysuria is a common complication of radical pelvic RT. Patients should be told to drink plenty and any infection should be treated with appropriate antibiotics. Anticholinergic drugs such as propantheline 15 mg t.d.s. or emepronium 200 mg t.d.d.s., may be helpful for troublesome frequency and nocturia. Symptoms may persist for some weeks or months after RT and occasionally bladder function never returns to normal.

Vaginal problems

Acute reactions in the vaginal mucosa are inevitable after radical pelvic RT, especially after intracavitary treatment. Arrangements should be made for patients to have saline douches regularly for a week or so after treatment. As the mucositis resolves vaginal adhesions occur and patients who wish to resume sexual intercourse should be counselled to start again as soon as possible using artificial lubricants, as dryness is a common and persistent problem. If vaginal stenosis does develop it may be helped by the use of graduated vaginal dilators.

It is not surprising that many patients experience problems with intercourse following radical pelvic RT. Dyspareunia is common because of adhesions, stenosis and dryness. Premenopausal patients will also have a RT-induced menopause which may exacerbate the problems, and there may be psychological difficulties related to the diagnosis of genital cancer that may lead to loss of libido. Patients should be warned of the potential problems and be questioned specifically but sympathetically during follow-up and appropriate advice given or referral made.

Central nervous system (CNS) syndromes

Headache, nausea and general malaise are quite common during RT to the brain and there are also two specific syndromes that occasionally occur during and soon after RT to the CNS:

L'hermitte's syndrome: 'electric-shock' paraesthesiae down the back of the legs, especially on neck flexion, can occur when lengths of the cervical and upper thoracic spinal cord are irradiated. It usually settles spontaneously without long-term sequelae after a month or so.

Somnolence syndrome: drowsiness and sometimes ataxia occurring during or a few weeks after high-dose cranial RT, especially in children. It is usually self-limiting.

3.7 Long-term problems after radiotherapy

Skin care

After radical RT with high dose at the skin surface, long-term changes occur. The skin tends to become thin and atrophic with abnormal pigmentation and telangiectasia and there may be areas of subcutaneous fibrosis. Eventually skin necrosis may occur especially after trauma. Patients should be advised to take particular care of these areas of skin, to avoid sunshine exposure (which may worsen RT damage) and trauma. Moisturizing creams may help to keep the skin supple and camouflage cosmetics may be needed for unslightly telangiectasia.

Biopsy should be avoided whenever possible.

If necrosis occurs, it should be managed like any other simple ulcer, but healing may be very slow. Skin grafting should be considered if no healing has occurred after a month of conservative measures.

Gastrointestinal problems

Changes in bowel habit, especially diarrhoea, are common after abdominal and pelvic RT. Usually reassurance and treatment with antidiarrhoeals and antispasmodics are sufficient, but persistent and severe symptoms (especially if associated with pain, subacute obstruction or weight loss) should prompt investigation to exclude tumour recurrence, fibrous adhesions or ulceration. High-dose RT to the rectal mucosa (e.g. from RT to prostate or cervix) may induce mucosal telangiectasia which can bleed easily. However, persistent bleeding should not be attributed to this without excluding a colonic tumour by sigmoidoscopy and barium enema. If telangiectasia is proven to be the cause, patients should be advised to take a high-residue diet or be given stool softeners. Severe and persistent rectal bleeding may rarely necessitate a colostomy.

Genitourinary problems
The kidneys are quite sensitive to RT (see Table 3.4) and so great care is usually taken not to irradiate them unless absolutely necessary. RT to one kidney may result in subsequent hypertension. If this is difficult to control, nephrectomy of the irradiated kidney may be needed.

Ureteric obstruction may be caused by RT fibrosis but is more usually due to tumour recurrence or nodal involvement.

High dose of RT to the bladder can produce bladder wall fibrosis and mucosal telangiectasia resulting in frequency, dysuria and haematuria. It is of course essential to exclude tumour recurrence by cystoscopy. Cystectomy and ileal conduit may be required for severe problems.

Lung problems
Radiation pneumonitis is a syndrome of dry cough, dyspnoea and infiltrative changes on chest X-ray in the irradiated area of lung, starting 2 or 3 months after RT. It is a self-limiting process which may be helped symptomatically by corticosteroids (e.g. prednisolone 10 mg t.d.s.) and usually results in an area of permanent fibrosis.

If X-ray changes do not conform to the RT portals other, infective, causes must be sought, especially in immunosuppressed patients (see section 4.3).

4   General management problems

4.1   Nutrition

Weight loss

This is a frequent problem in patients with malignant disease. It may be a result of advancing disease or a side-effect of treatment. Its causes are often multiple and ill-defined but it is important not to overlook potentially reversible factors.

   Weight loss may be caused by the following:
- inadequate food intake
- malabsorption
- altered metabolism
- fluid loss

Inadequate food intake

This is the major cause of weight loss and may result from one or more of the following:

1   Altered taste sensation: local effect from radiotherapy, chemotherapy or a remote tumour effect.

2   Dry mouth: local effect of radiotherapy, chemotherapy, other drugs (e.g. antihistamines, antidepressant, opiates).

3   Stomatitis (see section 3.6): local effect of radiotherapy, chemotherapy (especially methotrexate, adriamycin, bleomycin), oral candidiasis, herpes simplex, aphthous ulcers, iron and/or vitamin deficiency.

4   Dysphagia: mechanical obstruction from tumour, local effect of radiotherapy, neuromuscular causes.

5   Oesophagitis: local effect of radiotherapy, chemotherapy (especially adriamycin, bleomycin, methotrexate), candidiasis, herpes simplex. Remember that chemotherapy, especially adriamycin, may enhance radiotherapy-induced oesophagitis and vice versa.

6   Dyspepsia: peptic ulcer (drug-induced, e.g. steroids), oral chemotherapy, parenteral chemotherapy, gastric involvement by tumour.

7   Anorexia: depression, remote tumour effect, opiates.

8   Nausea and vomiting: drugs (especially cytotoxics, opiates),

4.1   Nutrition

hypercalcaemia (see section 4.7), uraemia, raised intracranial pressure (see section 4.8), intestinal obstruction (see section 4.2), ileus, abdominal radiotherapy (see section 3.6).

9 Abdominal disension: ascites (see section 4.2), tumour mass, hepatomegaly, splenomegaly, constipation.

Malabsorption

This is an uncommon cause of weight loss in patients with cancer but should be considered in certain situations as listed below:

• obstruction of the pancreatic duct (carcinoma of pancreas, portal node metastases)

• common bile duct obstruction (carcinoma of the pancreas, portal node metastases, cholangiocarcinoma)

• radiation to the bowel (producing stricture or fistula)

• bowel fistula

• blind loop syndrome

• intestinal resection

• carcinoid syndrome

• small bowel tumour (especially lymphoma with or without pre-existing coeliac disease)

• VIPoma

• chemotherapy (rare, e.g. methotrexate)

Altered metabolism

Several changes in metabolism have been described in patients with cancer. These include an increased basal metabolic rate, glucose intolerance, increased lipolysis and a negative nitrogen balance. The causes of these changes are unknown. It has been postulated that tumour products analogous to hormones are responsible.

Nutritional assessment

Regular *weighing* is essential in the management of patients with cancer. Changes in weight often correlate closely with the progress of the disease. They form a very useful and easy assessment of nutritional status but it should always be remembered that rapid change may be caused by changes in fluid balance (e.g. ascites, oedema).

Weight loss is also a frequent presenting symptom of cancer, and may be very substantial (1 stone weight loss represents roughly 10% of total body weight). Thus, *early* nutritional assessment and dietary advice is often very important.

Muscle mass
Measurement of mid-arm circumference and skin-fold thickness provides a useful index of nutritional status, but requires experienced personnel for consistency of measurement and is more applicable to clinical research than general clinical management.

Laboratory tests
Some useful tests for nutritional assessment are:
- serum albumin (most commonly used)
- 24-hour urea excretion
- thyroid-binding globulin
- serum transferrin

Nutritional support
Many patients will require dietary advice on nutritional support during the course of their disease and its treatment.

Nutritional support does not appear to reverse severe cachexia from advanced cancer, but may improve the patient's general well-being, and tolerance of intensive chemotherapy or radiotherapy.

Nutritional support takes three main forms:
- dietary advice and supplements
- enteral feeding
- parenteral feeding

Dietary advice and supplements
Anorexia and nausea are frequently encountered in patients with cancer, associated with the disease or its treatment. Management of these symptoms is difficult and they often do not resolve until treatment is discontinued or the disease responds. Anorexia may be

improved with steroids and if depression is present, antidepressants may help. A wide range of anti-emetic drugs is available to control nausea (see section 4.2).

A dietician is invaluable in taking an accurate dietary history and in giving detailed and specific advice on problems such as dysphagia and constipation. In addition, advice on the most appropriate dietary supplements can be given.

Some useful hints to anorectic patients include:
● eat little and often
● avoid the smell of cooking
● eat food which you like (this seems obvious but many patients may feel that foods which they particularly like are 'bad' for them)
● supplement meals (see below)

Many dietary supplements are available, some of which are available on prescription. There are two main types:

Energy supplements — comprising concentrated carbohydrate. They may cause osmotic diarrhoea, and are not nutritionally complete (see Hycal, Maxijul). They are frequently unpalatable but can be incorporated into other foods.

Complete supplements — these contain most necessary nutrients and are usually fairly palatable. They do not generally cause osmotic diarrhoea (e.g. Fresubin, Ensure). Their appropriate use requires the help of a dietician.

Cancer diets
Several alternative medicine and 'cancer help' centres now recommend 'cancer diets' which they believe may modify the progress of malignant disease. There is no evidence to support the use of such diets but many patients are eager to try them. Many are strict vegetarian or even vegan diets, requiring vitamin supplements, and many patients find them difficult to tolerate. Weight loss is common on such diets. Although these diets may help patients to feel that they are making a positive contribution towards their treatment, their use cannot be recommended.

4 General management problems

Many booklets concerning dietary information are currently available for patients. The booklet produced by BACUP (see appendix 6) is one example.

Enteral tube feeding
Tube feeding is very useful in patients who are unable to eat, either because of intractable nausea, or because of mechanical/neuromuscular problems in the mouth, oropharynx or upper GI tract. It is clearly of no benefit in patients who have malabsorption. It should usually be considered only when there is a reasonable chance of cure or significant palliation from treatment.

Indications:
• mechanical obstruction of the upper GI tract (e.g. carcinoma of the head and neck)
• dysphagia from other causes (e.g. neuromuscular)
• severe stomatitis or oesophagitis
• severe anorexia

Several systems are now available with fine-bore nasogastric tubes, often complete with bottles and giving sets. Most systems incorporate reverse Luer locks to prevent accidental i.v. infusion of enteral feeds.

Insertion requires care to ensure correct positioning of the tube. There is a possibility of accidental insertion into the right main bronchus without producing discomfort to the patient. It is therefore *essential* to check the position of the tube with a chest and plain abdominal X-ray after insertion.

A number of complete feeds are available for enteral use with fine-bore systems. In the absence of evidence of malabsorption, feeds containing nitrogen as whole protein rather than oligopeptides or free amino acids are preferable. For most adult patients who are not severely catabolic, a regimen comprising 3 litres of fluid, 2000–3000 calories and about 10 g of nitrogen per day is satisfactory, although this will sometimes have to be individualized.

Feeds are ideally given by continuous drip over 24 hours, but for a patient at home, feeds can be given as 4–6 aliquots, or given in 12 hours overnight.

4.1   Nutrition

Common complications of tube feeding are:
- blockage of the tube — especially with fine-bore systems
- tube regurgitation or accidental removal
- ulceration and stricture (very rare with fine-bore tubes)
- insertion of the tube into airways
- osmotic diarrhoea
- abdominal pain or bloating
- hyperglycaemia
- hypoleukaemia

Regular weighing, full blood counts, urea and electrolytes and liver function tests are essential during tube feeding.

Provided patients and their relatives have adequate motivation and support, enteral feeding can be managed at home.

Parenteral nutrition

This should be considered for patients in whom enteral tube feeding is not appropriate, either because of malabsorption or because of inability to tolerate a nasogastric tube. Many patients who are having intensive combination chemotherapy will have a tunnelled subclavian line already *in situ* and if they require nutritional support, then this route should be used.

Parenteral nutrition should only be considered in patients who need short-term nutritional support during a period of crisis and when there is a reasonable chance of returning to normal feeding, because the treatment is expensive, complex and difficult to discontinue once started. Parenteral nutrition must be given into a large central vein,preferably the superior vena cava. A tunnelled subclavian line is preferable since this will reduce the risk of line infection (see section 5.4 for care of tunnelled lines).

Regimens for parenteral nutrition are beyond the scope of this chapter. They vary according to individual patients and centres. The nutrition should always be supervised by experienced medical and nursing staff.

Common complications of parenteral nutrition include:
- line-related infection
- fluid overload

4 General management problems

4.1 Nutrition

- hyperglycaemia
- trace element, vitamin and electrolyte deficiency (although most regimens now incorporate trace elements and vitamins)
- disturbed liver function (elevated transaminases and alkaline phosphatase)

4.2 Gastrointestinal problems

Nausea and vomiting
These may be related to the presence of cancer but are more commonly encountered as a toxic effect of treatment.

Causes
Disease-related
- intestinal obstruction
- upper GI tract tumours — due to a direct local effect, or by producing obstruction
- massive abdominal distension — ascites or tumour
- raised intracranial pressure
- metabolic causes, e.g. hypercalcaemia, uraemia
- liver metastases

Treatment related
- cytotoxic drugs — especially cisplatin, mustine, nitrosoureas and dacarbazine (DTIC)
- opiate analgesics
- radiotherapy of, for example, whole abdomen, pelvis and whole brain

Anti-emetics
Numerous anti-emetics are available. No single anti-emetic regimen is clearly superior and regimens therefore vary enormously between centres. In addition, a major problem with patients receiving repeated courses of chemotherapy is 'anticipatory' nausea and vomiting, which can be intractable.

For patients receiving non cisplatin-based chemotherapy, the following anti-emetics are frequently used:

- prochlorperazine
  5–10 mg orally 4- to 8-hourly or 25 mg suppository 4-hourly
- metoclopramide
  10–20 mg orally 4-hourly or 10 mg i.v. 4- to 6-hourly
- domperidone
  10–20 mg orally 4- to 6-hourly or 30–60 mg suppository 8-hourly

For cisplatin-based chemotherapy, commonly used additional drugs include:

- dexamethasone
  8 to 10 mg i.v. at time of treatment and 4 hours later $\pm$ 10 mg orally on night before chemotherapy
- lorazepam
  2–4 mg on night before chemotherapy and 2–4 mg i.v. at time of chemotherapy $\pm$ 2 mg orally on night before chemotherapy

It is important to remember that antiemetic drugs have unwanted side-effects such as drowsiness and extrapyramidal syndromes.

Mouth ulceration

Ulceration of the mucous membranes is uncommon except when anticancer treatment has been used. Host-tissue factors and poor oral hygiene may also make patients susceptible to oral ulceration. Treatment-related factors include radiation and drug therapy (especially methotrexate, adriamycin).

General treatment

Prophylaxis is very important and all patients at risk should be taught to use regular antiseptic mouth washes (e.g. chlorhexidine) and brush their teeth regularly with a soft tooth-brush or to use cotton wool-tipped swabs. Mouth washes should not contain alcohol.

Pain is a major problem, especially at meal times. Viscous lignocaine paste can be used for temporary pain relief. Cocaine mouth washes may also be helpful, as may soluble aspirin gargles. If pain is very severe, it is sometimes appropriate to use anaesthetic mouth washes (e.g. Difflam) or even opiate analgesics.

In severe cases vigorous cleaning and removal of exudate is necessary, with opiate analgesic cover. Hydrogen peroxide mouthwashes are very useful for removing exudate.

If ulceration or monilial infection develops, remove exudate before treatment and give intensive antifungal agents. General care is of paramount importance. As soon as drug-related neutropenia recovers, the monilia also usually improves.

Chemotherapy-induced oral ulceration
Anticancer drugs damage the rapidly dividing cells of the normal mucous membrane. Ulceration usually appears about 5 days after treatment and lasts 4–10 days. The severity of the effect can vary, from pain without loss of mucosal integrity, to total loss of the mucous membrane of the mouth. The condition can be further complicated by superinfection with monilia (see below). Drugs which commonly cause mucosal ulceration include:
- methotrexate
- adriamycin
- bleomycin

Although folinic acid mouth washes may be of use in methotrexate-induced ulceration, no specific treatment for other drugs is available and supportive care, plus good oral hygiene, is the only treatment commonly available.

Radiotherapy-induced oral ulceration (see section 3.6)

Monilial infection
Monilial ulceration is a frequent problem. The typical appearance is of a white creamy exudate or an ulcerated base. This may be patchy, or in severe cases involves nearly the whole of the nasopharynx. Infection of the oesophagus is quite common and may cause dysphagia. A barium swallow or oesophagoscopy will help diagnostically.

Specific treatment
This comprises intensive use of one of the following antifungal agents:
• nystatin lozenges or suspension (100 000 units in 1 ml) 2- to 4-hourly
• nystatin pastilles — sucked continuously
• amphotericin B lozenges — kept against buccal mucosa but not sucked continuously
• ketoconazole tablets or suspension 200 mg b.d. (amphotericin should be discontinued if ketoconazole is used because of potential interactions)

Herpes simplex may cause mouth ulceration also and should be considered in patients receiving intensive chemotherapy, especially if the patient has cold sores around the mouth. Appearances are non-specific and a trial of oral acyclovir 200 mg, 5 times daily may be appropriate.

Diarrhoea
This can be caused by the tumour itself, its treatment, or occasionally by infections. Before starting treatment to relieve diarrhoea it is important to be sure that the patient does not have faecal retention with overflow (do a rectal examination).

If the diarrhoea is directly caused by the tumour, then specific antitumour therapy is the most logical approach to its control. Diarrhoea is a common side-effect of pelvic radiotherapy and certain drugs, but this can usually be controlled readily. Common treatment-related causes of diarrhoea are:
• broad-spectrum antibiotics
• radiotherapy (see section 3.6)
• chemotherapy — methotrexate, 5-fluorouracil, cisplatin, cytosine arabinoside
• infection

Specific treatment
• surgery, radiotherapy or chemotherapy as indicated

• pancreatic enzyme replacement for steatorrhoea caused by carcinoma of the pancreas

General treatment
Common antidiarrhoeal treatments are:
• codeine phosphate tablets 30–60 mg 4–6 hourly
• diphenoxylate with atropine (Lomotil) 1–2 tablets 4 times a day
• loperamide 1 to 2 capsules 3–4 times a day

Constipation
Many patients with cancer complain of constipation. This may be a direct effect of the tumour, or hypercalcaemia, in which case antitumour therapy is of major importance. Drugs are however the commonest cause of constipation in cancer patients. The most important drug-induced causes of constipation are the use of:
• opiate analgesics
• vinca alkaloids

Treatment
The treatment of constipation, apart from that due to intestinal obstruction, is the judicious use of aperients. The 2 main types are:
• stool softeners — liquid paraffin, lactulose, methyl cellulose, dioctyl sodium sulphosuccinate
• purgatives — e.g. bisacodyl, senna
   Most patients do best with a combination of both types of aperients. Enemata and manual evacuation are also quite frequently necessary for severe constipation and suppositories may also help. In patients receiving opiate analgesics, aperients should be given routinely as prophylaxis.

Ascites
This is a frequent and troublesome problem in cancer patients. The common causes include:
• widespread tumour involvement of the peritoneum (e.g. ovarian carcinoma, lymphoma) causing malignant ascites

• distortion or rupture of the thoracic duct (especially in lymphoma) causing chylous ascites
• liver failure
• severe hypoalbuminaemia

Management
• confirm the diagnosis and its cause — an ultrasound may be helpful as may a diagnostic tap for biochemistry, bacteriology and cytology
• symptomatic relief can be obtained by paracentesis
• diuretics will help ascites due to liver failure and hypoalbumin-aemia, and occasionally malignant ascites
• systemic chemotherapy for responsive tumours (e.g. lymphomas)

Paracentesis is a simple and relatively safe technique which can be readily repeated in patients with malignant ascites. Remember the following points:
• confirm by clinical examination or ultrasound that abdominal swelling is not due to massive tumour or intestinal obstruction.
• a peritoneal dialysis catheter can be used and is usually quite comfortable
• avoid obvious tumour masses, possible distended bowel and old scars
• drain ascites slowly (no more than 1 litre immediately and 1 litre per hour thereafter); rapid drainage may cause hypotension and collapse
• if drainage continues after 24 hours remove catheter because the rate of production of ascites is rapid — further drainage will produce hypovolaemia and hypoalbuminaemia, and will increase the risk of infection

Intestinal obstruction
This is a common presentation of colonic tumours and is often a feature of ovarian and other pelvic tumours, although it may also be produced by post-operative and post-radiotherapy adhesions. At

presentation, the management of intestinal obstruction is almost invariably surgical, usually involving either resection or bypass of the obstructing lesion. This may be followed by radiotherapy or chemotherapy if the underlying tumour is likely to respond.

Recurrent ovarian carcinoma presents particular problems since tumour is often widespread within the peritoneal cavity, involving multiple loops of bowel. This often causes a typical and insidious onset of subacute intestinal obstruction, sometimes with minimal signs and without classic radiological features. Many patients have features of an ileus because diffuse involvement of the bowel interrupts autonomic pathways. Because of the widespread involvement, surgery is not always possible or desirable, although a surgical opinion should usually be sought. Chemotherapy offers some chance of palliation, but temporary relief can be obtained from nasogastric tube drainage and intravenous fluids.

In patients with terminal disease and complete intestinal obstruction a nasogastric tube may relieve vomiting but can be uncomfortable. With judicious use of anti-emetics and opiates it should be possible to keep patients comfortable and vomiting to a minimum for several days without resort to nasogastric drainage.

4.3 Infection in cancer patients

All cancer patients are at a greater than normal risk of developing infections. Generally, their investigation and treatment should be the same as for patients without malignant disease. Patients who are receiving intensive chemotherapy causing prolonged neutropenia and those with haematological malignancies are especially vulnerable, and require particular advice and management.

Prophylaxis for patients having chemotherapy

Strict avoidance of all possible sources of infection in the community is an unnecessary (and impossible!) restriction for most patients on chemotherapy. However, they should be advised to avoid individuals with obvious infectious illnesses such as measles or chickenpox.

4.3   Infection in cancer patients

Most bacterial infections are endogenous, arising from colonizing organisms. The hospital environment is heavily contaminated with pathogens and infection may be transferred from staff, catheters, air, foci of bacterial contamination in the ward, and food. So, a neutropenic patient who is otherwise well is probably safer at home but requires clear instructions to contact the hospital if he becomes unwell or develops a fever.

Isolation rooms are not necessary, except for specialized procedures such as high-dose chemotherapy with bone marrow transplantation, and/or patients with acute myeloid leukaemia undergoing intensive remission induction chemotherapy because of the prolonged period of marrow depression. Even for these cases, complete isolation with barrier nursing is unnecessary. Simple measures to prevent cross-infection (e.g. single room, hand washing) are usually adequate.

Mouth care is important in all patients receiving chemotherapy, especially when neutropenic (see section 4.2).

Focal sepsis may occur, particularly affecting the skin and perineum, and is a particular problem with:

• i.v. catheter sites — peripheral venous catheters should be checked routinely for signs of infection. Routine re-siting of cannulae is probably unnecessary as long as sites are regularly inspected. Tunnelled central venous cannulae must also be inspected daily.

• urinary catheters — these are a major source of infection and should be avoided whenever possible

All invasive procedures (e.g. blood sampling, drip siting) require *strict* aseptic technique.

Prophylactic antibiotics and antifungals

In general these are unnecessary and potentially dangerous because of the possible development of resistant organisms. Their use should be restricted to patients who are likely to undergo periods of prolonged immunosuppression following chemotherapy. Examples include patients treated for:

- acute lymphoblastic leukaemia
- non-Hodgkin's lymphoma (treated with high-dose chemotherapy)
- patients receiving high-dose chemotherapy with bone marrow transplantation

Prophylaxis should be considered in those patients who are at risk of developing the following:

- *Pneumocystis carinii* — co-trimoxazole has proven prophylactic value at a dose of 4 tablets 3 times weekly
- candidiasis — oral ketoconazole (200 mg daily) as well as oral nystatin should be considered although its value is as yet unproven

Prophylaxis against viral infections
Viral infections which commonly occur in the immunosuppressed are generally not preventable, except by avoidance of exposure. The following infections should now be avoidable by screening of blood products:

Cytomegalovirus (CMV). This can cause severe pneumonitis and hepatitis. Patients who are to receive intensely immunosuppressive chemotherapy and numerous blood products should have their CMV antibody levels determined before starting therapy. If antibody levels do not indicate previous exposure, these patients should receive screened CMV-negative blood products to reduce their risk of infection. For patients who have detectable antibody, these precautions are pointless and screened blood is not required.

Acquired immune deficiency syndrome (AIDS). All blood products are now screened for human immunodeficiency virus (HIV).

Immunization
This is not available for any of the infections which commonly cause problems in immunosuppressed patients and, in those most at risk, the likelihood of an adequate immune response to the vaccine is small.

Patients on chemotherapy or those with lymphomas or leukaemias should only receive killed vaccines. A certificate of exemption should be given where a live vaccine is required for travel to certain countries. However, patients should be strongly advised not to travel to such countries whilst receiving treatment.

Killed vaccines	Live vaccines
polio (Salk)	polio (Sabin)
influenza	measles
typhoid	yellow fever
paratyphoid	rubella
cholera	

Diagnosis of infection

Non-neutropenic patients (neutrophils $\geqslant 1.0 \times 10^9$/litre)
A source of infection will usually be apparent in this group and investigations can be directed towards the most likely focus.

Neutropenic patients (neutrophils $< 1.0 \times 10^9$/litre)
If neutropenic patients have a documented fever of 38°C or over, or if they give a strong history of fever and rigors but have no fever when initially seen, urgent investigation and treatment are essential.

These patients can deteriorate extremely quickly and may look reasonably well until a few minutes prior to circulatory collapse.

While an accurate diagnosis of infection in this group is desirable, it is rarely possible, and it is safer to start treatment after appropriate investigation, and review the patient frequently.

Antibiotic treatment should be started as soon as appropriate cultures have been taken, but before the results are available.

Investigations
• a thorough clinical examination may indicate a source of infection (remember that neutropenic patients are unable to form pus, and a focus of infection may not be evident), e.g. i.v. cannulae, local skin sepsis, perineal infection, dental sepsis

81

• blood cultures — these should be taken from a peripheral vein and also through a central venous catheter if present
• throat swab
• MSU
• chest X-ray
• 10 ml serum for subsequent viral/bacterial/protozoal antibody screen

It should be remembered that there are other causes of fever; examples include:
• underlying tumour (lymphoma, sarcoma)
• drugs (e.g. bleomycin)
• transfusion of blood products

Treatment of bacterial infections

Non-neutropenic patients
These patients should be treated in the standard way. If an obvious source of infection is present it should be treated appropriately.

Neutropenic patients
Gram-negative bacteraemia is a common problem in this group of patients. Parenteral administration of two bactericidal antibiotics with a broad-spectrum is standard treatment. The standard combination is with an aminoglycoside (e.g. gentamicin, amikacin) and a broad-spectrum pencillin with significant anti-*Pseudomonas* activity (e.g. azlocillin, piperacillin, ticarcillin). In cases of penicillin allergy, a cephalosporin can be substituted (e.g. cefuroxime, cefotaxime). Gentamicin should be avoided when cisplatin has been recently (within 28 days) administered because the nephrotoxicity (and ototoxicity) of both drugs may be enhanced.

Several studies now support the use of single broad-spectrum antibiotics for neutropenic fever (e.g. ciprofloxacin, ceftazidime). However, further data are required from randomized studies before this can be regarded as standard treatment.

Other antibiotics may be added to the standard combination

depending on clinical circumstances. Examples include:
- metronidazole — for dental infections, perineal infections, anal fissures, etc.
- cloxacillin — where staphylococcal infection is likely — paronychia, skin sepsis, tunnelled line infection, i.v. cannula infection
- vancomycin — for central i.v. cannula infections due to *Staphylococcus epidermidis* (although such cannulae should be removed if a line-related fever does not settle rapidly on antibiotics)

The minimum duration of antibiotic therapy should be 5 days, or until the white cell count improves and the patient is afebrile. If the patient has prolonged neutropenia, antibiotics may be discontinued if he or she remains afebrile for 7 days, but the patient should remain in hospital until the white cell count recovers.

Treatment of fungal infections

Local fungal infections
Mucocutaneous candidiasis often occurs in the following patients:
- those on corticosteroids
- those receiving chemotherapy
- patients with Hodgkin's disease or non-Hodgkin's lymphoma
- patients with mucositis due to drugs or radiotherapy
- patients with severe cachexia

It most commonly affects the mouth (see section 4.2) but infection may spread to the oesophagus and stomach, causing severe dysphagia. The diagnosis of oesophageal candidiasis requires endoscopy or a barium swallow. Vaginal candidiasis may also occur in these patients, and candida may produce balanitis in men.

Treatment of oral candidiasis is covered in section 4.2.

Oesophageal candidiasis should be treated with ketoconazole 200 mg 5 times daily which can be given in syrup form for patients with dysphagia. Amphotericin lozenges should not be used in conjunction with ketoconazole since there is a potential interaction between the two. Vaginal candidiasis can be treated with preparations such as clotrimazole which is available in pessary and cream formulations.

Systemic fungal infections

Systemic fungal infection should be seriously considered if a high pyrexia persists for more than 5 days in spite of adequate antimicrobial therapy, if cultures are repeatedly negative, and if the patient's condition is deteriorating. The optimum duration of treatment is controversial but probably less than the 6-week period frequently advised. Standard treatment is with intravenous amphotericin, which is toxic, especially to the kidneys. It should be given as follows:

- take fungal blood cultures
- give a 1 mg test dose of drug, covered with 10 mg chlorpheniramine i.v. and 100 mg hydrocortisone i.v.
- if this is tolerated start at 0.5 mg/kg daily given by a 4-hour infusion, also covered with chlorpheniramine and hydrocortisone
- if condition fails to improve, increase dose by 0.25 mg/kg per day to a maximum dose of 1 mg/kg per day
- monitor renal function and electrolytes (especially K^+, Mg^2+ and creatinine) daily
- continue treatment for at least 7 days or until white cell count recovers

Meningeal fungal infections such as *Candida albicans* and *Listeria* should be treated with systemic antifungal agents. Although rarely used, intrathecal amphotericin can be given to seriously ill patients.

Cryptococcal meningitis

Headache may be present but fever and a gradually deteriorating mental state are common. Lumbar puncture is diagnostic — the test for cryptococcal antigen is specific and sensitive. Treatment is with intravenous amphotericin, with or without intrathecal treatment.

4.3   Infection in cancer patients

Viral infections
Viral infections are probably more common in immunosuppressed patients than is realized, and undoubtedly account for some febrile episodes which appear to respond to antibiotics, and some which do not.

Herpes virus infection is the commonest clinical problem. The most important forms of herpes virus infection are:

Herpes simplex — classic 'cold sores' may spread to produce severe peri-oral and oral ulceration. The diagnosis should be considered if oral ulcers fail to resolve with usual measures (section 4.2). Genital herpes simplex may produce an ulcerative vulvitis or balanitis.

Herpes zoster — this may take the form of classic dermatomal herpes zoster, but in the immunocompromised patient, may present as, or progress to disseminated herpes zoster, which is often severe and life-threatening.

Management is as follows:
- take vesicle fluid or swab into virus transport medium for electron microscopy
- take blood for viral antibody titres
- herpes simplex oral and perineal lesions — give topical and oral acyclovir (200 mg 5 times daily for 7 days)
- herpes zoster dermatomal lesions — therapy is only indicated if new lesions are developing — give i.v. acyclovir 10 mg/kg t.d.s. for at least 5 days; monitor renal function
- disseminated varicella zoster — give i.v. acyclovir 10 mg/kg t.d.s. for at least 7 days.

Cytomegalovirus (CMV) presents with fever, malaise and frequently evidence of abnormal liver function. Treatment is symptomatic, although a new agent, gancyclovir, is undergoing trials at present and may shortly become available generally.

Protozoal infections
These infections are relatively rare, but life-threatening and a high
index of clinical suspicion is required. The three principle forms
affecting cancer patients are:

Pneumocystis carinii
Rapidly progressive dyspnoea and cough, frequently associated
with widespread pulmonary shadows or chest X-ray characterize
the infection. Patients with defects of cell-mediated immunity (e.g.
Hodgkin's disease) are especially at risk. Prophylaxis should be
considered in patients at particularly high risk during chemotherapy
including those with:
- acute lymphoblastic leukaemia
- lymphoblastic lymphoma
- Hodgkin's disease
- non-Hodgkin's lymphoma treated with intensive chemotherapy
- patients undergoing high-dose chemotherapy with autologous
bone marrow rescue.

Prophylaxis is with co-trimaxozole one tablet b.d. throughout
chemotherapy and for at least 3 months after.

For suspected infection the following measures should be taken:
- take blood for *Pneumocystis* antibody titres
- transbronchial biopsy or bronchial lavage should be performed in
an attempt to make the diagnosis histologically (although if this is
not possible it may be necessary to treat empirically)
- treatment should be with high-dose co-trimoxazole — 4 tablets
q.d.s.
- if there is no response to co-trimoxazole, consider pentamidine (in
which case histological confirmation of the diagnosis is essential)

Cryptosporidium
This is a protozoan parasite which causes a self-limiting diarrhoeal
illness in the healthy, but life-threatening debilitating diarrhoea and
vomiting in immunosuppressed patients (e.g. AIDS, patients receiving chemotherapy). The diagnosis is made by identification of

oocysts in the stools of infected patients. Treatment is largely supportive including antidiarrhoeals, anti-emetics and intensive nutritional support. Steroid therapy should be discontinued if possible. Spiramycin may improve symptoms, although its value in eradicating the organism is unclear.

Toxoplasma gondii
Severe disseminated infection involving the heart, brain, liver and kidneys can occur. The treatment is pyrimethamine 25 mg daily for 4 weeks.

4.4   Respiratory problems

Dyspnoea
This is the most common symptom and may be due to:
- infection — viral, bacterial, fungal or protozoal
- pulmonary embolism
- anaemia
- pleural effusion
- lymphangitis
- large airway obstruction
- pain, e.g. metastatic involvement or fracture of rib
- drug induced pulmonary fibrosis, e.g. bleomycin
- drug-induced pulmonary fibrosis, e.g. bleomycin
- radiation-induced pneumonitis (see section 3.7)
- anxiety states
- other medical conditions (e.g. heart failure, asthma)

Remember that a chest X-ray may be normal despite underlying bronchospasm, chronic bronchitis and emphysema, small metastases, miliary TB, early interstitial pneumonia and acute pulmonary embolism. Treat the underlying condition and give oxygen if indicated. Severe dyspnoea in terminally ill patients is best controlled by opiates.

Chronic cough
If due to primary tumour or pulmonary metastases, this can often be suppressed with codeine linctus, or if severe, a small dose of opiate (e.g. diamorphine).

Haemoptysis
This may be due to a primary tumour, metastasis or pulmonary infarction. It is not a common feature of thrombocytopenia although it may be confused with epistaxis in which blood may be seen at the back of the nasopharynx. Chronic cough may produce a slightly blood-stained sputum. Blood loss is rarely severe and episodes usually subside spontaneously. Radiotherapy is usually the treatment of choice, although chemotherapy may be used where a rapid response can be anticipated (e.g. small cell carcinoma of the bronchus). Severe haemoptysis as a terminal event may be due to erosion of a major vessel and is best managed by sedation. Platelets should be given for thrombocytopenia.

Stridor
This can be caused by large airway obstruction by tumours of the pharynx and larynx, lung, oesophagus or by gross mediastinal lymphadenopathy (e.g. lymphomas). It is very distressing and frightening for patients when severe, and requires urgent treatment as follows:
- 35% oxygen
- consider tracheostomy for upper airway obstruction
- urgent radiotherapy
- chemotherapy if the tumour is likely to be very chemosensitive (e.g. lymphoma)
- dexamethasone 4 mg q.d.s.
- bronchoscopic laser therapy for tracheal tumours

Lymphangitis carcinomatosa
This is caused by diffuse infiltration of pulmonary lymphatics by tumour, especially carcinoma of the breast or lung. It is usually

bilateral, and associated with progressive dyspnoea and a dry cough. If the underlying tumour is responsive, chemotherapy should be used. Steroids may provide some symptomatic relief.

Pleural effusions
These are common in cancer patients and may present as dyspnoea, cough or pain. Infection and infarction are common causes in addition to malignancy. Management is as follows:
• diagnostic aspiration — send for protein, glucose, culture, ZN stain and cytology
• therapeutic aspiration — this should be performed if there is respiratory embarrassment
• no more than 1500 ml should be removed at a single aspiration because of the risk of pulmonary oedema
    The subsequent treatment includes:
• treatment of the underlying malignancy — if the underlying tumour is chemosensitive, commence systemic treatment
• for recurrent effusions attempt chemical pleuredesis with tetracycline (see section 5.12)

Pulmonary embolism
This is a common cause of death in patients with cancer, partly due to the underlying tumour, and partly as a result of debility and immobility. The decision to anticoagulate cancer patients should be made in the light of their likely long-term prognosis. Any underlying cause of the venous thrombosis (e.g. inferior vena cava compression) must also be treated. Confirmation of the diagnosis by ventilation-perfusion scan or venograms is essential before starting anticoagulation.
    Thrombocytopenia is a relative, but not necessarily absolute, contraindication to full anticoagulation.

Radiation pneumonitis
See chapter 3.

4.4   Respiratory problems

Drug-induced pneumonitis
The chemotherapeutic agents which most commonly produce pneumonitis are bleomycin, busulphan, cyclophosphamide and methotrexate. Diffuse infiltrative shadows are most commonly seen on chest X-ray, although nodular or pleural shadowing may occasionally occur. The changes may be progressive and produce a restrictive ventilatory defect.

Methotrexate can produce fine recticular shadowing but symptoms are rarely severe. High concentrations of oxygen are thought to potentiate bleomycin-induced pulmonary fibrosis and this must be borne in mind if the patient requires a general anaesthetic.

The changes are usually irreversible. Treatment comprises:
• discontinuing the drug
• steroids may be of some benefit

Tuberculosis
Reactivation of TB can occur in any patient who has malignant disease and should always be considered where there is immuno-suppression. It should be remembered in the following situations:
• prolonged pyrexia of unknown origin
• lack of response to antibiotics
• pancytopenia
• alcoholism or diabetes mellitus
• Hodgkin's disease and non-Hodgkin's lymphoma
• the elderly
• patients with chest X-rays showing old tuberculosis changes
In some high-risk patients — such as those treated for TB previously — who are receiving chemotherapy, chest radiotherapy or high-dose steroids, prophylaxis should be considered and discussed with a chest physician.

4.5   Cardiovascular problems

Heart failure
Many patients with cancer are middle-aged and elderly and have a

high incidence of overt or asymptomatic ischaemic heart disease. They are therefore at risk of developing heart failure. Common precipitating factors are:
- anaemia — due to bleeding, haemolysis or bone marrow suppression
- fluid overload during chemotherapy, e.g. hydration for cisplatin
- fluid retention due to corticosteroids
- cardiomyopathy — drug-induced (adriamycin, daunorubicin and high-dose cyclophosphamide)
- arrhythmias
- tumour involvement of the pericardium with tamponade
- tumour involvement of the myocardium, e.g. bronchial and breast carcinomas, lymphomas
- renal failure

Heart failure should be treated conventionally. The underlying cause must also be treated.

Dysrrhythmias
These can be precipitated by:
- drugs (adriamycin, daunorubicin)
- pericardial involvement by tumour
- myocardial involvement by tumour
- metabolic disturbances secondary to the malignancy or its treatment

Treatment is conventional, again with attention towards the underlying cause.

Superior vena cava obstruction
Compression of the SVC is most commonly caused by:
- bronchial carcinoma
- non-Hodgkin's lymphoma
- Hodgkin's disease
- teratoma

The clinical features are:
- headache

4.5   Cardiovascular problems

- swelling of the neck, face and hands
- fixed elevation of jugular vein pulse (JVP)
- suffused conjunctivae
- papilloedema and retinal venous engorgement
- increasing dyspnoea
- rarely, stridor due to laryngeal oedema

If SVC obstruction occurs in a patient with an established diagnosis, management is:

- radiotherapy, or
- chemotherapy — for tumours which are likely to respond rapidly, e.g. small cell lung cancer, lymphoma; do *not* inject drugs into arm veins if they do not collapse on elevation
- steroids have been extensively used but are of doubtful benefit

In patients who present with superior vena cava obstruction without an established diagnosis, a diagnosis should be searched for exhaustively before therapy is started, since this may hinder subsequent investigation.

Signs of SVC obstruction may not resolve following chemotherapy or radiotherapy since thrombosis frequently occurs, and it may not recanalize. Recurrent SVC obstruction is difficult to treat and indicates a poor prognosis. Opiates may help to relieve distress.

Pericardial effusion and tamponade
Asymptomatic pericardial effusions are fairly common in cancer patients, although tamponade is rare.

The most common cause is direct tumour involvement of the pericardium. The tumours most likely to cause an effusion are:

- bronchial carcinoma
- breast carcinoma
- lymphoma
- leukaemia

Clinical features
- increasing dyspnoea
- pericardial pain

4.5   Cardiovascular problems

- dizziness
- tachycardia
- elevated JVP
- 'low cardiac output' state
- exaggerated pulsus paradoxus
- soft heart sounds and a rub
- enlarged nodular heart shadow on chest X-ray

Diagnosis
This should be confirmed by echocardiography.

Management
This is urgent and consists of:
- pericardial aspiration — by an experienced person, preferably under ultrasound guidance. Fluid should be sent for culture and cytology and a cannula can be left *in situ* for continuous drainage.
- radiotherapy
- chemotherapy for very chemosensitive tumours
- pericardial window for recurrent effusions

Thrombotic problems
Cancer patients have an increased incidence of venous thrombosis, both deep and superficial. This is probably in part a humoral effect of the tumour on coagulation (e.g. Trousseau's syndrome — flitting thrombophlebitis as a marker of otherwise occult internal malignancy).
Other causes include:
- retroperitoneal tumours
- pelvic tumours
- lymphadenopathy — especially iliac, inguinal, femoral
- oestrogens
- surgery
- immobility
- chemotherapy — *never* use foot or leg veins

Management
This is conventional, with support stockings, elevation and analgesics if necessary. The decision to anticoagulate must be based on
the likely long-term prognosis for the patient. Thrombocytopenia is
a relative, but not absolute contraindication to anticoagulation.

Pulmonary embolism
See section 4.4.

4.6   Haematological problems
Haematological complications are common in malignant disease,
either due to the underlying disease, or its treatment.

Bone marrow failure
This may be due to two distinct processes:
• bone marrow suppression, e.g. due to cytotoxic drugs or wide-
field radiotherapy
• bone marrow infiltration by malignant cells
The complications of both are similar, as is the supportive care, but
the treatment of the underlying cause is often quite different.
Distinction between the two processes depends on a number of
factors:
• the presence of known tumour in the bone marrow (although
sampling error can give a false negative result)
• the time scale of the fall in the blood count
• the relationship of the change in haemoglobin, white cell count,
and platelets to cycles of chemotherapy

Bone marrow suppression
The white cell count usually falls first after around 5–10 days
following chemotherapy, followed by the platelet count at 10–14
days and the haemoglobin at a much slower rate. Some drugs may
cause more prolonged bone marrow suppression (e.g. nitrosoureas,
carboplatin), and thrombocytopenia can occasionally persist for
weeks or even months. Slow release of methotrexate from a
reservoir site such as an effusion or cerebrospinal fluid (CSF) can

produce a similar effect, which is potentially very dangerous. Prolonged folinic acid rescue is necessary for patients with effusions or oedema. After prolonged chemotherapy marrow reserve is depleted and a given dose of drug will produce a greater degree of suppression. A hypoplastic or aplastic state may develop after prolonged chemotherapy, especially with alkylating agents.

Drug-induced acute myeloid leukaemia occurs in a small proportion of patients between 6 months and 10 years after treatment with alkylating agents or procarbazine.

Bone marrow infiltration

Thrombocytopenia is the commonest presenting feature of marrow infiltration by tumour. Quantification of the degree of infiltration is difficult, except in the leukaemias, because of the sampling error of bone marrow biopsies. Infiltration of the bone marrow by a solid tumour usually indicates a poor prognosis.

Where bone marrow infiltration is present, chemotherapy (or hormone therapy) is the only modality which is likely to be effective. As pancytopenia of variable degree is often present, the usual guidelines for dose reduction based on white blood cell and platelet counts do not apply. Haematological indices must be monitored carefully following chemotherapy since supportive care may be necessary.

Anaemia

This is a common feature of cancer and arises through a variety of causes:
- blood loss
- infection
- bone marrow infiltration
- nutritional disturbance
- haemolysis
- renal failure
- bone marrow depression
- 'anaemia of disseminated malignancy'

4.6   Haematological problems

Blood loss
This produces an iron-deficiency anaemia. If iron-deficiency anaemia is present at the outset in a patient with a solid tumour, blood loss is the most likely cause. Investigation of iron-deficiency anaemia is outside the scope of this chapter.

Infection
Chronic infection may be an important factor in some tumours such as lung cancer and tumours causing disturbance in the urinary tract (e.g. bladder, cervix).

Bone marrow infiltration
The anaemia is frequently leucoerythroblastic (with immature red and white cells in the peripheral blood).

Poor nutritional status
This can be caused in numerous ways (see section 4.1) and may contribute to the development of anaemia by impairing intake and reducing absorption of iron and other important haematinics.

Haemolysis
Acquired haemolytic anaemia is an uncommon complication of malignancy which usually occurs in lymphomas and leukaemias. Microangiopathic haemolytic anaemia may occur in carcinoma of the stomach, pancreas, prostate and with metastatic disease in bone.

Renal failure
This occurs frequently in malignancy although its contribution to anaemia is probably not very significant.

'Anaemia of disseminated malignancy'
This appears to result from impaired red cell production and increased destruction, for reasons which are poorly understood. It is usually normocytic and normochromic.

Treatment
The most effective treatment of all these types of anaemia is to control the underlying tumour when possible. Transfusion should be reserved for those patients who are symptomatic from their anaemia, or who are unlikely (e.g. because of chemotherapy) to reverse their anaemia without support. Transfusion is not without problems (hepatitis, hypersensitivity, fluid overload) and these should be balanced against the potential benefit. Packed red cells are usually preferable to whole blood. Occasionally patients who are sensitized to multiple HLA or white blood cell antigens may need washed or frozen red cells.

Iron and vitamin supplements are not generally of great use, unless there is a documented deficiency.

Neutropenia (see also section 4.3)
This is the commonest haematological side-effect of chemotherapy, usually developing within 5–10 days of treatment, and lasting for about 1 week. It is always reversible, but the risk of injection is considerable when the granulocyte count is below 10^9/litre (see section 4.3). Prophylactic antibiotics have no proven role. Some hospitals use sterile environments and regimens to sterilize the skin and gut. These measures have not been shown to improve infection rates or survival and can be very unpleasant for the patient. Their use should be confined to special situations such as bone marrow transplantation.

Any patient developing a fever at any time when they may be neutropenic *must* have an urgent full blood count. If this shows a neutrophil count of less than 10^9/litre, i.v. antibiotics should be started after if the appropriate cultures have been taken (see section 4.3).

Granulocyte transfusions are of no proven benefit in neutropenic patients and their use cannot be recommended.

Thrombocytopenia
This usually accompanies neutropenia and is most commonly a

result of chemotherapy. Hypersplenism is another important cancer-related cause (especially with lymphomas). Rarer causes include disseminated intravascular coagulation (DIC) and idiopathic autoimmune thrombocytopenia.

Thrombocytopenia secondary to drug treatment is almost always reversible, but there is, of course, a risk of haemorrhage. Spontaneous bleeding commonly only occurs when the platelet count is less than 20×10^9/litre. Aspirin and alcohol may cause severe bleeding with higher platelet counts, as may anticoagulants — the use of which must be carefully monitored.

Patients with severe thrombocytopenia ($<20 \times 10^9$/litre) should be examined daily for fresh purpura or fundal haemorrhages. Urine should be tested for blood.

Indications for platelet transfusion are:
• obvious haemorrhage, if platelets $<20 \times 10^9$/litre
• fresh purpura and/or fundal haemorrhages
• prophylaxis where risk of bleeding is high and thrombocytopenia will be prolonged (e.g. acute myelogenous leukaemia induction)
• prior to transfusion of other blood products (e.g. packed red cells) — the additional red cells will dilute the patient's circulating platelets
• prior to surgery when platelets are low
• prophylaxis in cytopenic patients who are infected, when platelet concentration is likely to be high.

Thrombocytopenic patients needing surgery should have pre-operative platelet transfusion to achieve a platelet count of more than 100×10^9/litre.

If initial platelet transfusion (usually 6 units) fails to control haemorrhage in a thrombocytopenic patient, further platelets should be given until the bleeding stops. In mild cases, transfusions 24 hours apart will control the problem, but a platelet count must be repeated daily. Platelet transfusions should be covered with intravenous hydrocortisone and chlorpheniramine to minimize allergic reactions. Where many transfusions are likely to be required over a prolonged period (e.g. after bone marrow transplantation) HLA-compatible platelets are preferable.

Immune thrombocytopenia requires treatment of the underlying tumour, steroids, and sometimes, splenectomy. Hypersplenism may also require splenectomy or splenic radiotherapy.

Thrombosis (see sections 4.4 and 4.5)
Thrombotic phenomena have been recognized as a complication of cancer for many years. They have been reported in a variety of carcinomas including pancreas, stomach and lung, as well as chronic myeloid leukaemia and polycythaemia rubra vera.

Overall, about 1 in 8 patients with cancer have some thrombotic complications. The common problems are recurrent or migratory thrombophlebitis, pulmonary embolism, arterial embolization and non-bacterial thrombotic endocarditis.

The mechanism of thrombosis is unknown, although numerous coagulation disorders have been described, of which DIC is the most common. In DIC, an exaggerated haemostatic response to tissue injury is initiated, circulating thrombin is generalized and fibrin is formed. A detailed account of DIC is not appropriate here — if the diagnosis is suspected, haematological advice should be sought.

Major principles of management include:
- treatment of underlying tumour
- replacement of blood products
- heparin

Haemorrhage
This can be caused by numerous factors in patients with cancer, and the following should be looked for:
- history of a prior bleeding tendency
- recent drug therapy (especially cytotoxics, anticoagulants, steroids and non-steroidal anti-inflammatories)
- site of bleeding
- purpura/fundal haemorrhages
- signs of liver failure
  Laboratory tests should include:
- full blood count
- platelet count

• prothrombin time (PT), partial thromboplastin time (PTT), thrombin time (TT), fibrinogen and fibrin degradation products (FDP)
• LFTs (liver function tests), V and Es (blood urea and electrolytes)
• microbiology if infection is suspected

Treatment
This will depend on the cause. Local measures and blood transfusion are required initially. If haemorrhage is severe, fluid and blood replacement should be monitored using a central venous line.
   Specific treatments for particular causes include the following:
• acute promyelocytic leukaemia — chemotherapy, heparin and blood product replacement
• Waldenstrom's macroglobulinaemia — plasmapheresis
• thrombocytopenia secondary to marrow infiltration — chemotherapy
• hypersplenism — treatment of underlying tumour, splenectomy
• immune thrombocytopenia — steroids, splenectomy
• chemotherapy-related thrombocytopenia — platelet support
• severe haemoptysis — radiotherapy
• liver failure — vitamin K

Hyperviscosity states
There are three main causes of hyperviscosity states in cancer patients:
• hyperleucocytosis — in chronic myeloid leukaemia and occasionally in acute leukaemias
• paraproteinaemia — in myeloma
• macroglobulinaemia (IgM-secreting lymphoma)

Clinical features
These may develop insidiously. They include:
• dyspnoea
• lethargy and confusion progressing to coma
• purpura and bruising
• retinal haemorrhages

- white cell count $> 150 \times 10^9$/litre
- paraproteinaemia

Treatment
- cytotoxic chemotherapy with measures to prevent acute tumour lysis syndrome (see p. 104–5)
- severe cases may require leukapheresis
- for paraproteinaemia urgent plasma exchange is indicated if there is clinical evidence of hyperviscosity since chemotherapy will not produce a rapid fall in paraprotein.

   Red cell transfusion is contraindicated during the acute phase of hyperviscosity.

4.7   Metabolic problems

Hypercalcaemia
Hypercalcaemia is a common complication of advanced cancer and occurs in haematological malignancies as well as solid tumours. It is particularly common in metastatic breast cancer (10–25% incidence). Remember that the calcium must be corrected for albumin, and a normal total calcium may represent hypercalcaemia in an unwell patient with hypoalbuminaemia. If unchecked, a cycle of dehydration, pre-renal and then intrinsic renal failure may develop.
Symptoms:
- thirst, with dry mouth
- lethargy and weakness, progressing to stupor or coma
- loss of appetite, nausea and vomiting
- polyuria and dehydration
- constipation
   Pathogenesis:
- metastatic bone disease (especially breast cancer, myeloma)
- ectopic hormone production (e.g. squamous cell carcinoma of the bronchus)
- ectopic osteoclast activating factor (OAF) in lymphoma, myeloma
- other medical causes — which should always be remembered

Treatment
This depends on the calcium level and the condition of the patient.
For mild elevations in asymptomatic patients oral hydration and
treatment of the underlying tumour is all that is needed. The
importance of the treatment of the malignancy itself cannot be over-
emphasized — all other measures to correct the hypercalcaemia are
of temporary benefit only.

First-line treatment involves the following:
• hydration — all symptomatic patients are dehydrated and
prompt, vigorous intravenous hydration is the most important factor
in the restoration of adequate renal function; normal saline should be
used as sodium and calcium excretion parallel each other; 3–4 litres
of fluid should be given daily, with careful monitoring of fluid balance
• steroids such as prednisolone are essential for tumours which are
intrinsically steroid-sensitive (e.g. lymphoma and myeloma), but are
of little benefit for other tumours
• diuretics — frusemide may promote calcium excretion once
adequate hydration has been restored.

If hypercalcaemia is resistant to these measures, consider:
• calcitonin — 3–8 MRC units/kg; this rapidly inhibits bone
resorption, but the effect is short-lived.
• mithramycin — this inhibits osteoblast activity and is useful for
resistant hypercalcaemia. The inhibition of bone resorption starts
within about 6 hours and lasts 4–5 days. An injection of 25 mg/kg
will often lower the calcium and may need to be repeated after 48
hours. It can be used chronically every 3–7 days, at the risk of some
toxicity, though the control of hypercalcaemia rarely lasts more than
7–10 days, but the main aim of treatment should be to control the
underlying tumour
• oral inorganic phosphate — may be used for choice treatment,
although it may cause diarrhoea
• diphosphonates — these are a new group of agents which are
effective for both short- and long-term management of malignant
hypercalcaemia: disodium etidronate and disodium pamidronate are
examples. The dosing schedules vary and are still undergoing

evaluation

• dialysis — this will temporarily lower the serum calcium but should only be considered when the renal function will not allow a forced diuresis, and when the underlying tumour is likely to be responsive to treatment; it is rarely needed

Hypocalcaemia

Symptomatic hypocalcaemia is uncommon. Cancer-related causes include:

• PTH deficiency — surgical removal of parathyroid glands or their destruction by tumour

• chemotherapy — mithramycin, cisplatin

• extensive osteoblastic activity in bony secondaries (e.g. carcinoma of breast or prostate)

Treatment

• check for hypomagnesaemia and correct — the calcium will otherwise be resistant to correction

• oral calcium supplements

• occasionally i.v. calcium chloride if symptomatic

Acute renal failure

The following are the important causes of acute renal failure in cancer patients:

• obstructive uropathy — extrarenal obstruction is common and may be caused by retroperitoneal lymph nodes (lymphoma, testicular tumours), retroperitoneal tumours (sarcoma), and pelvic tumours (ovary, cervix, bladder)

• hypercalcaemia (see above)

• paraproteins — associated with multiple myeloma and lymphomas; the resulting renal damage may be made worse by dehydration

• other tumour products (see below)

• direct renal infiltration by tumours — this is rare, but occasionally

seen with lymphoma or leukaemia
- direct toxic effects of therapy
    (i) cytotoxic drugs — especially cisplatin, where nephrotoxicity can be reduced by intensive hydration; other drugs include methotrexate and streptozotocin
    (ii) radiation nephritis (see section 3.5)
    (iii) antimicrobial and antifungal agents — complications are caused by aminoglycosides (which should not be used concurrently with cisplatin), cephalosporins and amphotericin

Management
As well as the general medical management of acute renal failure, specific measures may be required depending on the underlying cause:

Extrarenal obstruction
Abdominal ultrasound is the investigation of choice to make this diagnosis. Intravenous or retrograde pyelography are rarely needed. Treatment depends on the type of underlying tumour. Chemosensitive tumours such as lymphoma or teratoma can be readily treated and the renal failure is usually rapidly reversed. Radiotherapy may also be used for retroperitoneal or pelvic tumours. Unresponsive tumours may require nephrostomies or ureteral diversion, but in the face of disseminated incurable cancer, a relatively pain-free death from renal failure may be considered acceptable.

Paraproteins
Mild renal failure from paraproteinaemia is common in multiple myeloma, although acute renal failure is uncommon. Dehydration is a predisposing factor and is potentially reversible. Plasmapheresis may be indicated for severe renal failure.

Urate nephropathy and acute tumour lysis syndrome
Urate nephropathy is a potential problem with some chemosensitive tumours, particularly leukaemias and non-Hodgkin's lymphomas,

especially when tumour load is high. It can be prevented by the use of allopurinol 300 mg daily (or less if renal impairment exists), which should be commenced routinely in all such patients. If allopurinol sensitivity exists, probenecid can be substituted.

Acute tumour lysis syndrome may be a problem in patients with exquisitely chemosensitive tumours, particularly:

- acute leukaemias (with high initial white cell counts)
- lymphoblastic lymphomas
- Burkitt's or Burkitt-type lymphomas

Profound metabolic disturbances caused by massive tumour cell destruction can occur within a few hours of chemotherapy, including:

- hypercalcaemia
- elevated urea and creatinine
- hyperphosphataemia
- hypocalcaemia
- hyperuricaemia

Management includes:

- start allopurinol before chemotherapy
- intravenous hydration to ensure a diuresis of at least 100 ml/hour
- urinary alkalinization with oral sodium bicarbonate — to achieve a urinary pH of 7 or more and thereby normalize the urate level *before* chemotherapy; alkalinization should be discontinued once chemotherapy commences
- oral or rectal calcium resonium will reduce potassium absorption from the gut

Electrolytes, calcium, phosphate or urate must be closely monitored for at least 48 hours after chemotherapy. If the metabolic disturbance becomes severe, haemodialysis should be considered.

Drug-related renal failure

The important drugs are listed here:

- cisplatin — prehydration with intravenous saline, with or without mannitol, diminishes the nephrotoxicity of cisplatin, but renal impairment is still a problem with repeated treatments. In patients

who have renal impairment, the less nephrotoxic cisplatin analogue, carboplatin, can be used. Other potentially nephrotoxic drugs (e.g. gentamicin) should not be used with cisplatin
• methotrexate — when high doses are used with folinic acid rescue, the methotrexate may precipitate out in the kidneys. This can be prevented with vigorous hydration and urinary alkalinization to increase methotrexate solubility (see section 5.6). If nephrotoxicity develops, methotrexate clearance is reduced and prolonged folinic acid rescue is required. Methotrexate levels must be monitored when very high doses are used
• streptozotocin — this may cause a temporary rise in plasma urea, proteinuria or severe tubular damage with Fanconi's syndrome. Stop the drug and await recovery. If the damage is mild and recovery rapid, the drug may be restarted.

Hyperkalaemia
Hyperkalaemia may be life-threatening, causing depression of cardiac conduction, ventricular fibrillation or asystole, weakness, paralysis and ileus. In addition to the common medical causes, it may be caused by tumour lysis (see p.104).
   Treatment of hyperkalaemia is designed to correct acidosis, shift potassium into cells quickly, increase potassium excretion and treat the underlying cause.
   Emergency treatment consists of:
• infusion of 50 ml of 50% dextrose i.v. with 10 units soluble insulin
• infusion of 7 mmol calcium chloride i.v.
• infusion of 44 mmol sodium bicarbonate i.v.
• calcium resonium orally or as an enema
• monitor response by ECG, serum potassium and arterial blood gases for bicarbonate

Hyponatraemia
Inappropriate ADH secretion is a well-recognized problem in some cancer patients. It is characterized by hypo-osmolality, normovolaemia, normal renal function, less than maximally dilute urine

and appreciable urinary sodium excretion. Clinically it is characterized by weakness and lethargy, and in more severe cases, drowsiness, confusion and coma.

Most common tumour-related causes include:
- carcinoma of bronchus (especially small cell)
- bronchial carcinoid

and very rare causes are:
- adenocarcinoma of pancreas
- thymoma
- mesothelioma
- carcinoma of larynx
- leukaemias
- non-Hodgkin's lymphoma
- Hodgkin's disease
- CNS metastases
- drugs (vincristine, cyclophosphamide)

Diagnosis
Measure simultaneous serum and urine osmolalities.

Treatment
- control the underlying tumour
- fluid restriction (usually 1 litre/day) may restore osmolality to normal
- hypertonic saline infusions may help, although they produce volume expansion and hypo-osmolality may return
- demeclocycline can partially inhibit the action of ADH

(initially 900 mg–1200 mg daily in divided doses then 900 mg–900 mg daily)

4.8   Neurological problems
Neurological problems often present diagnostic difficulties in cancer patients since there are many possible causes:
- many tumours metastasize to the CNS with a variety of clinical presentations

- some tumours (especially bronchial carcinomas) produce non-metastatic effects on the CNS — 'paraneoplastic syndromes' (see p. 113)
- immunosuppressed patients may develop meningitis with unusual organisms or atypical symptoms
- tumours cause metabolic disturbances which may affect the CNS
- treatment may produce neurological symptoms (e.g. vinca alkaloid neuropathy, radiation myelitis)
- many cancer patients are elderly and at risk from cerebrovascular disease

Raised intracranial pressure
Classic symptoms are morning headache, nausea and projectile vomiting but these are often absent, particularly if the onset is insidious. The most reliable clinical sign is papilloedema though this may be absent with a slowly progressive lesion. In a patient known to have cancer an intracranial metastasis is the most likely diagnosis. This should, ideally be confirmed by a CT scan. If meningism is present a lumbar puncture should only be performed when a space-occupying lesion has been excluded. Treatment is urgent, especially if there are signs of brainstem or cerebellar dysfunction or deteriorating visual acuity. It consists of:

- reducing cerebral oedema: dexamethasone 4 mg p.o. 6-hourly (i.v. dexamethasone or mannitol are useful if a rapid response is needed)
- treat the symptoms — analgesics, anti-emetics
- treat the underlying cause (see below)

Cerebral metastases
These are most common in patients with bronchial, breast and renal carcinomas, malignant melanoma and some lymphomas. They may present in various ways including:

- raised intracranial pressure
- focal neurological signs
- fits

- meningitis

   The diagnosis should be confirmed by CT or isotope scan, or if there is meningism (with mass lesion excluded by CT), by lumbar puncture.

Treatment

- dexamethasone — up to 4 mg 6-hourly will reduce cerebral oedema and the symptoms of raised intracranial pressure, and may improve neurological deficit
- whole brain irradiation is the treatment of choice but should not be undertaken if the overall prognosis is poor
- systemic chemotherapy may be effective for chemosensitive tumours
- intrathecal chemotherapy (see section 5.10) — may be effective for meningeal involvement
- surgical excision — should only be considered when there is an isolated brain metastasis in a patient with no other evidence of disease and in whom the overall prognosis is good

Spinal cord compression

This is an emergency as progression can be rapid and the resulting neurological deficit irreversible. If the diagnosis is suspected, myelography should be undertaken urgently, preferably in a neuro-surgical centre, where emergency decompression can be carried out if the patient deteriorates during the procedure. At the time of myelography CSF can be taken for cytology, biochemistry and microbiology.

   Bone metastases with collapse or extradural deposits are the most common cause, usually from primaries in the breast, lung or prostate, or from lymphoma. Pain is a common presenting symptom and can be present for months before the first clinical sign. It is frequently useful for locating the metastases if the neurological signs are equivocal. If local tenderness is present an X-ray or bone scan may demonstrate a vertebral deposit.

4.8   Neurological problems

Management of suspected spinal cord compression
- careful clinical examination, looking for sensory level (remember saddle anaesthesia in cauda equina lesions)
- X-ray relevant part of spine, as suggested by clinical signs and any local bony tenderness
- if obvious vertebral collapse at appropriate level (usually several vertebrae higher than the top of the sensory level) and a histological diagnosis already established:

   start dexamethasone 4 mg q.d.s.

   nurse *flat*

   refer for *urgent* radiotherapy

   consider chemotherapy for very chemosensitive tumours (e.g. lymphoma, teratoma)
- if no obvious vertebral collapse, and/or no histological diagnosis refer for neurosurgical opinion and myelography
- if myelography is positive, surgical exploration is indicated, followed by radiotherapy or chemotherapy

Differential diagnosis
- non-metastatic syndrome
- radiation myelitis
- malignant meningitis
- non-cancer related causes (e.g. multiple sclerosis)

Meningitis
In the cancer patient presenting with signs and symptoms of meningitis, the differential diagnosis is:
- infection (bacterial, viral, protozoal)
- metastasis
- haemorrhage (especially in thrombocytopenic patients)

   Tumour infiltration of the meninges is common in leukaemia and lymphomas but rare in most carcinomas. Clinical features may include:
- multiple cranial nerve palsies
- extensive radicular disease

- signs of raised intracranial pressure
- meningism and photophobia
- pyrexia
- transverse myelitis

The diagnosis is made by lumbar puncture. CSF samples should be sent for:

- biochemistry — sugar and protein
- microscopy and culture
- cytology
- virology

The glucose is commonly reduced and the protein elevated. Abnormal cells may be present in the cytocentrifuge preparation. If no abnormal cells are seen but meningeal disease is suspected it is worth taking several samples. In cases of lymphoma the CSF should be examined for surface lymphocyte markers.

Treatment of leukaemic or lymphomatous meningeal involvement comprises intrathecal drugs — commonly methotrexate and cytosine arabinoside. Meningeal carcinomatosis rarely responds to intrathecal drugs. Cranial irradiation can be given concurrently with intrathecal chemotherapy or deferred until a response is seen. Infective causes of meningitis should be treated in the standard manner. Always remember tuberculosis as a possible cause of meningitis. Cryptococcal menigitis has an insidious onset and the diagnosis may require several lumbar punctures (see section 4.3).

Nerve, plexus and root involvement
Direct infiltration of peripheral nerves, plexuses or nerve roots can occur in many tumours. The initial symptom is normally pain, followed by a loss of motion and sensory function. Involvement of nerves and plexuses is usually by direct growth from primary and secondary tumours, and of nerve roots by meningeal tumours.

Common patterns of involvement include:

Cranial nerves
- head and neck tumours

- orbital tumours
- skull metastases (especially base of skull)
- lymphomas

Brachial plexus
- supraclavicular node involvement, e.g. lymphoma, bronchial and breast carcinoma
- apical lung tumour (Pancoast)

Sacral plexus
- retroperitoneal tumours
- pelvic tumours (e.g. cervix, bladder, lymphoma)

Nerve roots
- multiple — lymphoma, leukaemia
- individual — multiple metastases (e.g. myeloma, breast cancer)

Peripheral nerves (rare)
- diffuse — lymphoma, leukaemia
- individual — growth from any adjacent tumour

Treatment
The usual treatment of choice is local radiotherapy, but widespread involvement with leukaemia or lymphoma may respond to chemotherapy.

Peripheral neuropathy
This should be carefully distinguished by clinical examination from spinal cord compression, individual nerve involvement, or root/plexus involvement. In cancer patients, peripheral neuropathy is most often drug induced (see section 5.2) but may be a remote tumour effect (see paraneoplastic syndromes below).

The drugs most commonly responsible are:
- vinca alkaloids (which may also produce autonomic neuropathy and cranial nerve palsies)

- cisplatin
- procarbazine
- hexamethylmelamine

Drug-induced neuropathy usually recovers slowly once the drug is discontinued, although recovery may be incomplete.

Myopathy

The commonest cause of true myopathy in cancer patients is prolonged corticosteroid therapy. Myopathy may be part of a paraneoplastic syndrome.

Paraneoplastic syndromes

Some tumours, especially bronchial carcinoma, are associated with non-metastatic neurological dysfunction — paraneoplastic syndromes. The cause of these syndromes is unknown. They include:

- peripheral neuropathy — characteristically a segmental demyelination
- myaesthenic syndrome (Eaton – Lambert)
- subacute cerebellar degeneration
- transverse myelopathy

Treatment is that of the underlying tumour, following which there is sometimes improvement of the neurological syndrome.

Fits

These are commonly grand mal fits but may be Jacksonian where a localized space-occupying lesion is present. Immediate anticonvulsant therapy should be used, with standard drugs. The following causes should always be considered:

- intracerebral tumour
- meningeal infection
- meningeal tumour
- electrolyte abnormalities (e.g. low Ca, Mg)
- anoxia
- intracranial haemorrhage
- intracranial venous thrombosis
- drugs, e.g. cisplatin

Toxic confusional states

Symptoms may vary from a mild confusional state to deep coma. The following underlying causes should be considered:

- hypercalcaemia
- ectopic ADH production
- hyperglycaemia
- frontal lobe metastases
- encephalopathy
- cranial irradiation
- drug related (opiates and sedatives)
- infection (see section 4.3)
- hyperviscosity (see section 4.6)
- anoxia

Look for a treatable underlying cause. Treat the underlying tumour when this is justified by a good long-term prognosis. Patients with mild to moderate disorientation benefit from familiar surroundings and continuing of care.

4.9   Alopecia

Many cytotoxic drugs cause some degree of hair loss, in particular the anthracyclines and alkylating agents given intravenously in high doses (see section 5.2). Alopecia is therefore a very common problem, and often very distressing to the patient.

Radiotherapy causes localized alopecia within the field of treatment. The extent of regrowth is dose-dependent and is often incomplete after high-dose irradiation.

It is essential to reassure the patient that hair usually comes out gradually over a few weeks, starting 14–21 days after commencing chemotherapy or radiotherapy, rather than suddenly, and that it will grow again as soon as treatment is stopped. The regrown hair can vary in texture and colour from the original hair. Wigs are available on NHS prescription for patients receiving chemotherapy or cranial irradiation and these should be offered to the patient before alopecia is established. Wigs for women tend to be more cosmetically acceptable than those for men.

4.9   Alopecia

Attempts to reduce alopecia have included scalp cooling. This is rarely useful and can be uncomfortable and distressing. In addition there is a small risk that tumour cells in the scalp may receive less drug, such that scalp metastases may occur.

4.10 Pain control

Pain is a common, though by no means inevitable, symptom of malignant disease and therefore a frequent problem in management.

Causes

The first important step in the management of pain is to make an accurate diagnosis, since the pain may not necessarily be due to the tumour. It may be caused by one or more of the following:

Primary tumours

Direct involvement of:
- peripheral nerves
- nerve roots and plexuses
- spinal cord
- soft tissues
- viscus
- bone

Secondary effects of tumours

- inflammation and oedema
- infection
- obstruction
- pathological fracture
- raised intracranial pressure

Effects of treatment

- post-surgery (especially amputation, mastectomy, thoracotomy)
- chemotherapy-induced phlebitis and tissue damage
- peripheral neuropathy (vinca alkaloids, cisplatin)
- mucositis, oesophagitis (chemotherapy, radiotherapy)

4.10 Pain control
_____

- steroid withdrawal polyarthralgia
- steroid-induced peptic ulcer
- post-irradiation nerve plexus fibrosis, myelopathy or tissue necrosis

Other causes
- herpes zoster and post-herpetic neuralgia
- intercurrent illness
- intestinal obstruction

Management
The management depends on the underlying cause.

Surgery
This is useful in many situations:
- pinning pathological fractures in long bones
- bypass or removal of tumour obstruction
- relief of extradural compression of spinal cord or nerve roots

Radiotherapy
This is very useful in controlling pain due to local tumour infiltration (see section 3.4). It should always be considered unless the prognosis is very poor or the patient is too unwell to tolerate treatment.

Chemotherapy
This can often be used to relieve pain directly related to tumours. It is indicated when the tumour is likely to be chemosensitive or when radiotherapy is not possible, either because of the extent of the disease, or because of recurrence of tumour within a previously irradiated area.

Nerve blocks
Nerve blocks are useful when pain is due to direct infiltration of nerves, plexuses or roots. Of particular use are brachial plexus,

4.10 Pain control

intercostal and coeliac plexus blocks, as well as intrathecal nerve blocks. The usual procedure involves injection of neurolytic agents such as phenol, but analgesia of several weeks duration can be obtained from injections of local anaesthetic. The procedures require skill and are potentially hazardous and should be performed only by anaesthetists experienced in their use.

Analgesic drugs
These are obviously the mainstay of management of pain, but require careful choice and prescribing for maximum benefit and minimum toxicity. Before prescribing analgesics it is worth discussing the characteristics of the pain in considerable detail. One should elucidate the site, periodicity, quality, duration and severity of the pain as well as assessing the patient's psychological state, social support and awareness of the problem, and explain how the drugs will help.

Many patients worry about addiction to opiate analgesics or that the drugs will become less effective with more use, and they consequently tend to under-use drugs. Reassurance at this point is essential and it is important to explain that the purpose of the analgesic treatment is to keep the patient as free from pain as possible.

The most important principle of analgesic prescribing is regular administration to prevent pain occurring rather than giving analgesics only when pain occurs. For most drugs the length of effect is such that regular 4-hourly administration is needed (see below). In addition to their regular doses of analgesics, patients should be prescribed a reserve supply of a stronger analgesic or advised to take a larger dose any time there is a sudden exacerbation of pain.

As far as possible analgesics should be given orally and parenteral administration reserved for emergency relief of pain or when oral drugs cannot be tolerated, which should only be for a few days at most.

117

4.10 Pain control

Non-narcotic analgesics
These should be tried first in patients with mild pain:
- aspirin 300–1200 mg 4-hourly
- paracetamol 500–1000 mg 4-hourly

Aspirin may cause dyspepsia and gastrointestinal bleeding. Very high doses may cause tinnitus and hyperventilation. Either aspirin, or other non-steroidal anti-inflammatories such as indomethacin are particularly useful in the management of pain due to bony metastases, and may be used in conjunction with strong opiates.

There are numerous different formulations of these drugs and it is best to prescribe one or two with which one is familiar. If the pain is not well controlled by a non-narcotic drug of adequate dosage a weak narcotic should be given.

Weak narcotic analgesics
These should be used for controlling moderate pain and when non-narcotic drugs have failed. Useful drugs include:
- codeine 30–60 mg 4–hourly
- dihydrocodeine 30–60 mg 4-hourly

Both of these produce, to some extent, the side-effects of strong opiates (see below) but constipation is usually the most troublesome.

The combination of dextropropoxyphene/paracetamol (Distalgesic, Co-Proxamol) is very popular with patients and doctors but there is little evidence that the dextropropoxyphene contributes to the analgesic effect of the paracetamol at the dose used.

Strong narcotic analgesics
These are often required when other drugs fail. The most commonly used are morphine and diamorphine which are best given orally, 3- to 4-hourly. Morphine is also available in slow-release form (MST), and can therefore be given on an 8- or 12-hourly basis.

When oral analgesics are not tolerated, other analgesics include:
- morphine suppositories 10–20 mg
- diamorphine by injection — either s.c., i.m. or i.v.

4.10 Pain control

Continuous s.c. or i.v. infusions of diamorphine are very useful in patients with very severe, poorly controlled pain.

Side-effects of narcotics include:

- sedation — variable; tends to decrease with continued use
- nausea — tends to improve after 7–10 days; some patients may require regular anti-emetics
- constipation — almost inevitable; regular laxatives should be given
- addiction and tolerance — these are not a significant problem in patients with chronic pain
- respiratory depression

Phenothiazines

Drugs such as promazine and chlorpromazine may be used in some patients to potentiate the analgesic effect, suppress nausea and vomiting and increase sedation associated with narcotic analgesics.

4.11 Pregnancy and contraception

Pregnancy in a woman requiring treatment for malignant disease presents obvious problems. The management has to be individualized and requires much careful thought and discussion. In general, if systemic chemotherapy or abdominal radiotherapy is planned, therapeutic abortion should be advised for pregnancies in the first trimester. In the third trimester it may sometimes be possible to delay treatment until after delivery, which may be induced early if adequate neonatal care is available. In the middle trimester therapeutic abortion is often the most appropriate course, although in some circumstances, such as Hodgkin's disease, it may be possible to give radiotherapy above the diaphragm with minimal risk to the fetus.

All cytotoxic drugs are potentially teratogenic and women receiving them should therefore be advised to continue taking contraceptive measures.

Alkylating agent therapy can produce temporary or permanent infertility (see section 5.3), but this is unpredictable and patients should continue to take contraception measures. If menstrual function returns after chemotherapy, normal pregnancy may still take place and the risk of malformation is not increased. In general, it is recommended that female patients do not attempt to have a pregnancy until about 1 year after the end of chemotherapy, although this time period is somewhat arbitrary. Advice should always, of course, be influenced by the likelihood of recurrent tumour.

Male infertility is also a common, although unpredictable consequence of chemotherapy, particularly when prolonged courses of alkylating agent treatment are used (e.g. Hodgkin's disease). It can also occur following any course of radiotherapy when the testes receive a significant dose . Many males will be rendered azoospermic, but again should be strongly advised to continue with contraceptives.

Because of the risk of azoospermia, young men about to undergo chemotherapy or scrotal irradiation should be offered the opportunity to store their sperm. Unfortunately, oligospermia is a common consequence of malignant disease, and the patient should be advised that he may have inadequate sperm counts before chemotherapy.

4.12 Psychological problems

Psychological disturbances are very frequent in patients with malignant disease and a detailed discussion is beyond the scope of this chapter. Anxiety and/or depression are a common reaction to the illness or its treatment, although some patients do not require specific therapy apart from having their problems discussed and questions answered.

Major psychotic episodes are uncommon, but some patients become profoundly anxious and depressed and antidepressant or anxiolytic drugs may be necessary, as may psychiatric referral.

Depressive or psychotic states may be the result of a number of organic causes including:

• hypoxia

4.12 Psychological problems

- pyrexia
- anaemia
- hyperkalaemia
- uraemia
- liver failure
- inappropriate ADH secretion
- drugs, e.g. opiates, steroids
- brain metastases (especially frontal lobe)
- non-metastatic syndromes (e.g. lymphoma-related subacute parencephalitis)

4.13 Fungating tumours and fistulae

These are common problems in advanced malignant disease, especially with tumours of the head and neck, breast and female genital tract.

Surgery is the definitive treatment of first choice but is often not possible for technical reasons when tumours are advanced. Radiotherapy may be used in addition or when surgery is impossible and chemotherapy may be tried for responsive tumours.

Offensive smell is a common symptomatic problem. This can be helped by regular cleaning and dressing, using a standard antiseptic such as chlorhexidine or povidone–iodine. A short course of broad-spectrum antibiotics may be useful if there is deep infection in any area that cannot be cleaned, and metronidazole is indicated where there is a possibility of anaerobic infection. Vaginal discharge associated with fistula may be helped by metronidazole in addition to regular local cleansing.

The normal skin around external fistulae should be protected with a suitable barrier and excess discharge managed either with regularly changed dressings or a stoma bag.

5   Anticancer drugs

5 Anticancer drugs

Cytotoxic drugs generally have a low therapeutic ratio, therefore a thorough understanding of their safe administration and their potential toxicities is essential to good patient management. It is not within the scope of this book to recommend specific drugs or combinations for all tumours, as chemotherapy is often a controversial and, sometimes, experimental area. In Appendix 1 we have, however, listed a number of commonly used combinations, with appropriate references.

In the first two sections of this chapter the cytotoxic drugs are listed and described. Section 5.1 lists cytotoxic drugs and hormonal agents in alphabetical order of approved or most commonly used names. For each drug, information is given on the group to which the drug belongs, dosage, mode of administration, precautions, toxicity, storage, interactions and, where known, on its metabolism. *The information on dosage is necessarily only an approximate guide,* not precise prescribing information, as doses will vary with different combinations. Reference should always be made to the regimen employed.

In particular, *the upper dose levels of many drugs can be associated with severe toxicity* and should only be administered under the supervision of those experienced in their use.

Section 5.2 is a list of the most commonly encountered toxicities under body systems and the drugs causing them, with an approximate rating of frequency. Very rare toxicities or those reported but with a dubious relationship to the drug are not included.

5.1 Alphabetical list of cytotoxic and hormonal agents

Toxicity rating scale (in the absence of antidotes, e.g. anti-emetics for nausea):

   $++++$ inevitable

    $+++$ common

     $++$ infrequent

      $+$ rare

Doses are an approximate guide, not precise prescribing informa-

5.1   Alphabetical list of cytotoxic and hormonal agents

tion. Always consult the dosage recommended in the particular regimen. In general, the lower recommended doses are those used in drug combinations.

Actinomycin D (dactinomycin, Cosmegen Lyovac)

Group: antibiotic

Dosage

> 0.015 mg/kg per day for 3–6 days. Usual max. daily dose   0.6 mg/m^2

Administration

> i.v. bolus into fast-running N. saline infusion

Precautions

> Avoid extravasation

Toxicity

+ + + +   Tissue necrosis

> Phlebitis

  + + +   Nausea and vomiting

> Myelosuppression (nadir at 10–14 days; recovery 16–20 days)

> Mucositis

    +   Alopecia

> Radiation recall

Monitoring tests

> Full blood count and liver function tests

Metabolism and excretion

> 50–90% excreted in the bile, 10–20% in the urine (consider dose reduction for liver functional impairment)

Storage

> Powder — 0.5 mg vials, refrigerated, away from light
> Solution — refrigerated, 24 hours

5   Anticancer drugs

5.1   Alphabetical list of cytotoxic and hormonal agents

Adriamycin (doxorubicin, 14-hydroxydaunomycin)

Group: antibiotic
Dosage

40–70 mg/m^2, usually given as a single i.v. injection once every 3 weeks

May also be given weekly at a reduced dose.

Total dose should not exceed 450 mg/m^2

Administration

i.v. bolus into fast-running N. saline infusion

Precautions

Avoid extravasation

Avoid skin contact (wear gloves and goggles when preparing and injecting)

Dose reduction if abnormal liver function (see below)

Toxicity

+ + + + Tissue necrosis

Phlebitis (use fast-running drip)

Complete alopecia

+ + + Nausea and vomiting

Myelosuppression (nadir at 9–14 days; recovery 16–20 days)

Mucositis

Pigmentation

Urine appears red for up to 24 hours after injection

+ + Nail changes

Pyrexia/rigors

+ Cardiomyopathy — increasing incidence at total doses of greater than 450 mg/m^2

Monitoring tests

Full blood count and liver function tests

Check cumulative dose does not exceed 450 mg/m^2

Monitoring of cardiac function (e.g. radionuclide ejection fraction) recommended if this dose exceeded

5.1   Alphabetical list of cytotoxic and hormonal agents

Metabolism and excretion

> Enterohepatic: consider dose reduction or omission if liver function tests abnormal (Bilirubin 20–50 µmol/l 50% reduction, >50 µmol/l 75% reduction)

Storage

> Powder — 10 mg, 50 mg vials, refrigerated
> Solution — refrigerated, away from light, 48 hours

Aminoglutethimide (Orimeten)

Group: hormonal agent: anti-adrenal and aromatization blockade

Dosage

> 250 mg, t.d.s. or q.d.s. continuously together with hydrocortisone, 20 mg b.d.

Administration

> Orally, 250 mg tablets

Precautions

> Simultaneous glucocorticoid administration essential
>
> Discontinue in the event of intercurrent infection, trauma, etc.
>
> Increase dose slowly over 3–4 weeks when starting treatment, especially in elderly

Toxicity

> +++ Sedation (can be severe, especially in elderly — introduce drug slowly)
>
> Rash after 7–14 days (mild, usually transient, even if drug continued)
>
> Adrenal insufficiency (ensure adequate glucocorticoid replacement — add fluorocortisone, 0.1 mg alternate days, if necessary)

Monitoring test

> Urea and electrolytes, BP lying and standing
> Full blood count

5   Anticancer drugs

5.1   Alphabetical list of cytotoxic and hormonal agents

Storage

Room temperature

Amsacrine (Amsidine)

Group: miscellaneous
Dosage

90 mg/m^2 i.v. daily for 5 days

Administration

Drug + diluent diluted in 500 ml 5% dextrose and infused over 60–90 minutes

Precautions

Avoid contact with skin or eyes

Avoid extravasation

Do not give in presence of hypokalaemia

Toxicity

+ + + + Myelosuppression

+ + + Phlebitis

Nausea and vomiting

+ + Hepatotoxicity

Renal toxicity

Alopecia

+ Grand mal seizure

Cardiac arrhythmias (predominantly in hypokalaemic patients)

Monitoring tests

Full blood count

Urea and electrolytes

Liver function tests

Storage

75 mg ampoules + diluent

Solution should be protected from light and used within 8 hours

5   Anticancer drugs

Androgens

Group: hormonal agents

Drugs, dosage and administration

> *testosterone* (Sustanon 100 and 250) every 4 weeks, i.m.
>
> *nandrolone phenylpropionate* (Durabolin, 25 mg amp.; 25 mg, 50 mg syringes) 25–50 mg/week, i.m.
>
> *nandrolone decanoate* (Deca-Durabolin, 25 mg, 50 mg syringes; 25 mg, 50 mg, 100 mg amp.) 25–50 mg every 3 weeks, i.m.
>
> *oxymetholone* (Anapolon, 50 mg tab.) 50–100 mg/day, orally
>
> *drostanolone* (Masteril, 100 mg amp.) 300 mg/week, i.m.

Precautions

> Ensure i.m. injections not given i.v. or s.c.
>
> Contraindicated in severe renal failure or heart failure

Toxicity

$++++$ Virilization

$+++$ Nausea and vomiting

$++$ Oedema (mild)

> Intrahepatic cholestatic jaundice (testosterone and methyl derivatives only)

Storage

> See manufacturers literature for individual drugs

Asparaginase (Colaspase, Crasnitin)

Group: enzyme

Dosage

> Variable, e.g. 20 000 i.u./m^2 weekly or 4000 i.u./m^2 daily $\times$ 14

5   Anticancer drugs

5.1   Alphabetical list of cytotoxic and hormonal agents

Administration

      i.m. injection preferred as anaphylactic reactions rare

      i.m. injection in <2 ml N. saline

Precautions

      To prevent acute anaphylactic reactions, skin test with 0.1 ml solution (20 i.u.) before each course

      Observe for at least 1 hour after injection

Toxicity

  + + + Pyrexia and rigors

      Hypersensitivity (usually mild and controlled by anti-histamines)

      Hepatic (usually transient elevation of enzymes)

    + + Hyperglycaemia

      Nausea and vomiting

     + Renal dysfunction

      Encephalopathy (occasionally coma)

      Myelosuppression

Monitoring tests

      Full blood count, liver function tests

Storage

      Dry—refrigerated, 4 years; room temperature, 2 years

      Solution—refrigerated, 3 weeks

Interactions

      Vincristine, hypoglycaemic agents

Bleomycin (Blenoxane)

Group: antibiotic

Dosage

      Multiple schedules. May be given s.c., i.m., i.v. or intracavitary

      Total dosage should not exceed 500 mg but caution should be exercised at total dosages greater than 200 mg

5.1   Alphabetical list of cytotoxic and hormonal agents

Administration

        i.v. bolus in 5–10 ml water or N. saline

        i.m. ⎫
             ⎬ dissolved in 0.5–1 ml of 1% lignocaine
        s.c. ⎭

        intracavitary (see section 5.12)

Precautions

        Check total dose is less than 500 mg. Consider monitoring lung function and chest X-ray if dose exceeds 200 mg. Avoid high-concentration oxygen administration under   anaesthetic

Toxicity

 + + + + Erythema and pigmentation of skin

   + + + Pyrexia/rigors (starts 3–6 hours; may be prevented with antihistamines or corticosteroids)

        Hyperkeratosis

        Pneumonitis and pulmonary fibrosis (dose-limiting, exacerbated by oxygen administration)

        Nail changes

        Alopecia

        Mucositis

    + + Radiation recall

     + Nausea and vomiting

        Phlebitis

Monitoring tests

        Clinical examination of the respiratory system and chest X-ray. If lung function tests are used, carbon monoxide transfer is the most sensitive indicator of pulmonary toxicity. Do not use in the presence of significant renal impairment

Metabolism and excretion

        Renal excretion

Storage

        Powder — 3 mg, 15 mg amp., room temperature

        Solution — stable 24 hours at room temperature

5 Anticancer drugs

5.1 Alphabetical list of cytotoxic and hormonal agents

Busulphan (Myleran)

Group: alkylating agent
Dosage

> Continuously, 0.5–10 mg daily, according to FBC (full blood count)
> Intermittently, 50–250 mg, as a single dose

Precautions

> May cause prolonged myelosuppression

Administration

> Orally, 0.5 mg, 2 mg tablets

Toxicity

  ++++ Myelosuppression (nadir 2–4 weeks; recover 4–8 weeks)

    +++ Infertility and amenorrhoea

> Pigmentation

       + Gynaecomastia

> Cataracts
> Nausea and vomiting
> Pulmonary fibrosis
> Leukaemogenic

Monitoring tests

> Regular full blood count

Metabolism and excretion

> Excreted in the urine as methanesulphonic acid

Storage

> Room temperature

Carboplatin (Paraplatin)

Group: miscellaneous
Dosage

> 400 mg/m^2 i.v. as a single agent. Reduced doses should be used if patient heavily previously treated or in presence of renal impairment. Given at 4-weekly intervals

5.1 Alphabetical list of cytotoxic and hormonal agents

Administration

i.v. infusion over 15–60 minutes

Pre-hydration not necessary

Precautions

Check renal function

Toxicity

$+ + + +$ Myelosuppression

$+ +$ Nausea and vomiting

$+$ Nephrotoxicity

Neurotoxicity

Allergic reactions

Monitoring tests

Full blood count and serum creatinine

Metabolism and excretion

Renal excretion

Storage

150 mg vials. Store at room temperature. Use within 8 hours of reconstitution

Carmustine (BCNU, BiCNU)

Group: nitrosourea

Dosage

Up to 200 mg/m^2 i.m., every 6–8 weeks

Administration

i.v. infusion over 15–45 min in 100–250 ml 5% dextrose

Flush with N. saline

Precautions

Follow carefully the manufacturer's instructions for making solutions. Dissolve the powder in each vial in 3 ml of absolute alcohol followed by 27 ml sterile water. Discard any vials with oily deposit indicating overheating and decomposition

5.1 Alphabetical list of cytotoxic and hormonal agents

Toxicity
+ + + + Tissue necrosis

Nausea and vomiting (severe—lasts 6–8 hours)

Phlebitis (pain at injection site and up the vein—try infusion 5 ml of 0.5% lignocaine)

+ + + Myelosuppression (moderate to severe: nadir at 3–4 weeks; recovery by 5–7 weeks)

+ + Facial flushing (lasts up to 2 hours)

Hepatic (transient elevation of enzymes)

Monitoring tests

Full blood count

Storage

Dry—refrigerated, up to 2 years; never store at >27°C

Solution—use as soon as possible, do not store

Metabolism and excretion

Rapid biotransformation—slow urinary excretion of metabolites

Crosses to cerebrospinal fluid

Interactions

Cimetidine

Chlorambucil (Leukeran)

Group: alkylating agent

Dosage

5–10 mg, daily continuous treatment

Administration

Orally, 2 mg, 5 mg tablets

Toxicity
+ + + Myelosuppression

+ Nausea and vomiting

Indigestion

Infertility

Hepatic

5.1   Alphabetical list of cytotoxic and hormonal agents

> Skin rash
>
> Pulmonary
>
> Leukaemogenic

Metabolism and excretion

> Unknown, probably extensive metabolism and renal excretion of metabolites

Storage

> Room temperature

Cisplatin (Neoplatin, Platinex)

Group: miscellaneous

Dosage

> Given every 3 weeks either as
>
> **1** 50–100 mg/m^2 in a single dose or
>
> **2** 15–20 mg/m^2 daily × 5

Administration

> Initial hydration then i.v. infusion in 1–2 l N. saline or 5% dextrose, at a rate of 1 mg/min (see section 5.7)

Precautions

> Check renal function (serum creatinine, or creatinine clearance) before each course
>
> Establish diuresis of >150 ml/hour before administration, and maintain for 6 hours after—keep up i.v. fluids until oral fluids tolerated (see section 5.11)
>
> Use mannitol (not loop diuretics), to enhance diuresis

Toxicity

> + + + + Nausea and vomiting (severe, lasts 12–24 hours)
>
> + + + Ototoxicity
>
> Myelosuppression (nadir at 3 weeks; recovery by 4 weeks)
>
> Renal failure (check renal function; ensure diuresis)
>
> Diarrhoea
>
> Hypomagnesaemia (very common biochemically, rarely symptomatic)

5.1 Alphabetical list of cytotoxic and hormonal agents

++ Hypocalcaemia (rarely symptomatic)

Neuropathy

Fits

+ Papillitis

Monitoring tests

Full blood count, urea and electrolytes, creatinine clearance, audiometry

Metabolism and excretion

Excretion mainly renal (reduce dose or omit if renal function impaired)

Storage

Dry—refrigerated, away from light, 2 years

Solution—room temperature, 24 hours

Interactions

Gentamicin

Cyclophosphamide (Endoxana)

Group: alkylating agent

Dosage

50–200 mg orally, daily, or 300–1000 mg/m^2 i.v., every 3 weeks

Administration

i.v. bolus + N. saline flush

Orally 50 mg tablets

Precautions

Patients should increase fluid intake (>3 l/day) to avoid cystitis

Toxicity

++++ Myelosuppression (nadir 1–2 weeks; recovery by 3–5 weeks)

Alopecia

Sterility

Nausea and vomiting (especially with high doses i.v.)

Haemorrhagic cystitis (consider mesnuma; see section 5.8)

++ Mucositis
   Amenorrhoea
+ SIADH
   Pulmonary fibrosis
   Leukaemogenic

Monitoring tests
   Full blood count

Metabolism and excretion
   Activated in liver
   Renal excretion

Storage
   Tablets—room temperature
   Powder—100 mg, 200 mg, 500 mg, 1000 mg vials, room temperature
   Solution—refrigerated 24 hours

Cytarabine (Cytosar, Alexan)

Group: antimetabolite

Dosage
   Multiple schedules

Administration
   i.v. bolus + N. saline flush
   i.m.
   s.c. in 0.5 ml of diluent
   Intrathecal (see section 5.10)

Precautions
   Reduce dose if severe liver dysfunction

Toxicity
++++ Myelosuppression (nadir at 5–12 days; recovery at 14–16 days)
++ Nausea and vomiting
   Mucositis
   Diarrhoea
+ Facial flushing
   Abdominal pain

5.1   Alphabetical list of cytotoxic and hormonal agents

Monitoring tests
>   Full blood count

Metabolism and excretion
>   Metabolized in the liver to uracil arabinoside
>   90% excreted in the urine as this inactive metabolite

Storage
>   Powder—40, 100 and 500 mg vials, refrigerated
>   Solution—refrigerated 48 hours

Dacarbazine (DTIC, imidazole carboxamide)

Group: miscellaneous; alkylating agent (?)

Dosage
>   250 mg/m^2 daily $\times$ 5
>   or 850 mg/m^2 $\Big\}$ every 3–4 weeks

Administration
>   i.v. bolus in 10 ml N. saline over 1 min, with N. saline flush
>   i.v. infusion in 100–200 ml 5% dextrose or N. saline over 15–30 min, with flush

Precautions
>   Avoid exposure to light
>   Avoid extravasation

Toxicity
> $+ + + +$ Myelosuppression (nadir at 3–4 weeks)
>   Nausea and vomiting (severe, 1–12 hours)
> $+ + +$ Phlebitis
> $+ +$ Pyrexia/rigors (especially after large single dose, start *c.* day 7, lasts 7–21 days)
>   Tissue necrosis

Monitoring tests
>   Full blood count

Metabolism and excretion
>   Mainly hepatic

5.1   Alphabetical list of cytotoxic and hormonal agents

Storage

100, 200 mg vials

Dry—refrigerated, away from light, 4 months

Solution—200–500 ml/N. saline or 5% dextrose, avoid exposure to light, use as soon as possible

Daunorubicin (Rubidomycin, Daunomycin, Cerubidin)

Group: antibiotic

Dosage

1–3 mg/kg or 50–100 mg/m^2 given as a single injection once every 3 weeks. Total dose should not exceed 600 mg/m^2

Administration

i.v. bolus into fast-running N. saline infusion

Precautions

Avoid extravasation

Avoid skin contact (wear gloves and goggles when preparing and injecting)

Reduce dose if abnormal liver function (see below)

Toxicity

+ + + + Alopecia

Tissue necrosis

+ + + Phlebitis

Nausea and vomiting

Myelosuppression (nadir at 9–14 days; recovery 16–21 days)

Red urine for up to 24 hours after administration

Mucositis

+ + Cardiomyopathy — increasing risk after total dose of 600 mg/m^2

Monitoring tests

Full blood count and liver function tests

Check cumulative dose does not exceed 600 mg/m.^{2} If higher dose given monitor cardiac function using, e.g. radionuclide ejection fraction

5   Anticancer drugs

5.1   Alphabetical list of cytotoxic and hormonal agents

Epirubicin (Pharmorubicin)

Group: anthracycline
Dosage

$50-90$ mg/m^2 intravenously every 3 weeks

Administration

i.v. into side arm of fast-running N. saline infusion. Avoid presence of cardiac disease. Monitor cardiac function if total dose exceeds 1 g/m^2

Precautions

Avoid contact with skin or eyes

Dose reduction for abnormal liver function tests

Toxicity

$++++$ Myelosuppression

Alopecia

Phlebitis (use fast-running infusion)

$+++$ Nausea and vomiting

$++$ Mucositis

Thrombophlebitis

$+$ Cardiomyopathy

Monitoring test

Full blood count and liver function tests

Check cumulative dose does not exceed 1 g/m^2. If higher doses used monitor cardiac function (e.g. by radionuclide ejection fraction)

Metabolism and excretion

Hepatobiliary excretion. Consider dose reduction or omission if liver function abnormal (bilirubin $20-50$ μmol/l 50% reduction, >50 μmol/l 75% reduction)

Storage

Powder — 10, 20 and 50 mg vials

Solution — store in refrigerator, use within 24 hours, avoid exposure to direct light

5.1   Alphabetical list of cytotoxic and hormonal agents

Etoposide (VP16–213, Vepesid)

Group: epipodophyllotoxin
Dosage

> Variable schedules. Often given day 1, 3, 5 or days 1–5 i.v. at 21-day intervals
>
> Orally, twice i.v. dosage

Administration

> i.v. infusion in 250–500 mg N. saline (not 5% dextrose) over 30–45 min
>
> Orally 50/100 mg capsules

Precautions

> Avoid extravasation
>
> Avoid rapid infusion
>
> Do not dilute in 5% dextrose

Toxicity

> +++ Myelosuppression (nadir at 2 weeks; recovery by 3 weeks)
>
> Alopecia
>
> ++ Nausea and vomiting (with oral capsules +++)
>
> Hypotension (occurs only with rapid infusion)

Monitoring tests

> Full blood count

Metabolism and excretion

> Mainly excreted in urine, partly in bile

Storage

> Intact vials 100 mg — room temperature, avoid light, 3 years
>
> Capsules — room temperature, 2 years

Fluorouracil (Fluoro-uracil, Efudix)

Group: antimetabolite
Dosage

> Various schedules. A convenient one is 500–1000 mg/m^2 i.v. or orally, weekly

5.1   Alphabetical list of cytotoxic and hormonal agents

Administration
> i.v. bolus + N. saline flush
>
> Topical use as an ointment (see section 5.11)

Toxicity

+ + + Myelosuppression
> Pigmentation

+ + Nausea and vomiting
> Phlebitis
>
> Mucositis
>
> Diarrhoea

+ Alopecia
> Skin rash
>
> Cerebellar ataxia
>
> Malabsorption
>
> Ocular

Monitoring tests
> Full blood count

Metabolism and excretion
> Entero-hepatic circulation. Only 15% excreted by the
> kidney

Storage
> Stable at room temperature, may precipitate if refrigerated
>
> Supplied in 250 mg vials (5 ml), 250 mg capsules and as
> an ointment

Folinic acid (Calcium Leucovorin, citrovorum factor)

Group: vitamins

Dosage
> 15–30 mg (depending on methotrexate dose) 6-hourly
> for 12–48 hours, starting 24 hours after methotrexate

Administration
> Orally, 15 mg tablets
>
> i.m.

i.v. bolus injection

Indications

Used to 'rescue' bone marrow and mucosal surfaces from toxicity of methotrexate, especially after high-dose treatment or in the presence of renal failure. Ideally, monitor serum methotrexate levels and give folinic acid if levels greater than 10^{-3} M at 24 hours, 10^{-6} M at 48 hours and 10^{-7} M at 72 hours (see section 5.6)

Gonadotrophin-releasing hormone analogues

Group: hormonal agents

Drugs, dosage and administration

buserelin (Suprefact)

Injection 5.5 ml vial — 1 mg buserelin/ml

Nasal spray, metered spray 100 dose unit

Advanced prostatic cancer: 0.5 ml buserelin injection 8-hourly for 7 days, then intranasal spray, one dose into each nostril 6 times daily

goserelin (Zoladex)

Implant 3.6 mg in syringe applicator

Advanced prostatic cancer: one implant subcutaneously every 28 days

Precautions

Tumour 'flare' may occur due to increased testosterone secretion during first 7 days of therapy. Avoid these agents in presence of ureteric obstruction or incipient spinal cord compression

Toxicity

$+ + + +$ Hot flushes

$+ + +$ Impotence

$+ +$ Gynaecomastia

Monitoring tests

Serum testosterone levels

143

5   Anticancer drugs

5.1   Alphabetical list of cytotoxic and hormonal agents

Hydroxyurea (Hydrea)

Group: miscellaneous
Dosage

20–30 mg/kg, continuously, according to blood count or
80 mg/kg every third day

Administration

Orally, 500 mg capsules

Precautions

Hygroscopic, keep bottles tightly closed

Toxicity

+ + + Myelosuppression (nadir at 10 days)

+ Nausea and vomiting

Mucositis

Pigmentation

Nail changes

Monitoring tests

Full blood count

Metabolism and excretion

Mainly renal

Storage

Room temperature; tightly closed bottles with desiccant

Ifosfamide (Mitoxana)

Group: alkylating agent
Dosage

1000–5000 mg/m^2 i.v. every 3 weeks
500–1000 mg/m^2 per day × 5, every 3 weeks

Administration

i.v. infusion
i.v. bolus in at least 75 ml water or N. saline + N. saline
flush

Precautions

Ensure adequate hydration during and after therapy to

maintain high urine output and minimize urothelial toxicity. Ideally, maintain i.v. infusion for 24–48 hours

Use mesna (see section 5.8) to prevent cystitis

Toxicity

+ + + + Haemorrhagic cystitis. Use mesna (see section 5.8) and increase fluid intake

+ + + Nausea and vomiting

Alopecia

+ + Myelosuppression

Phlebitis

Encephalopathy

+ Sedation

Nephrotoxicity

Leukaemogenic

Monitoring tests

Full blood count

Metabolism and excretion

Activated by liver microsomal enzymes

Metabolites excreted in urine

Storage

Available in 500 mg, 1 g and 3 g vials. Stable, when refrigerated, for 5 years

Dilute in water for injection, consult pharmaceutical literature for details.

Stable, when diluted for 1 week at room temperature and 6 weeks under refrigeration

If diluted in common infusion vehicles stable for 7 days at room temperature but use within 8 hours because no bacteriostatic properties

Lomustine (CCNU)

Group: nitrosourea

Dosage

100–300 mg/m^2 every 6 weeks

5.1   Alphabetical list of cytotoxic and hormonal agents

Administration

Orally, 10 mg and 40 mg capsules

Precautions

Avoid giving more often than 6-weekly because of prolonged myelosuppression

Toxicity

+++ Myelosuppression (moderate to severe: nadir 3–5 weeks; recovery by 6–10 weeks)

Nausea and vomiting (can be severe, lasts 2–6 hours)

+ Alopecia

Monitoring tests

Full blood count

Metabolism and excretion

Liver metabolism and renal clearance. Fat soluble, crosses to cerebrospinal fluid

Storage

Room temperature, 2 years

Melphalan (A^{lk}eran, L-phenylalanine mustard, L-PAM)

Group: alkylating agent

Dosage

5 mg/m,^{2} daily $\times$ 5, every 6 weeks

15–40 mg/m^2 orally or i.v. every 6 weeks

Administration

Orally, 2 mg, 5 mg tablets i.v. bolus + N. saline flush

Precautions

Orally—ensure given with food

i.v. dilute each 100 mg vial with 1 ml of propranolol diluent (supplied) and then 9 ml of water for injection

Toxicity

+++ Myelosuppression (nadir at 21–28 days)

++ Nausea and vomiting

Amenorrhoea

5.1 Alphabetical list of cytotoxic and hormonal agents

Sterility
+ Cystitis
Mucositis
Leukaemogenic

Monitoring tests

Full blood count

Metabolism and excretion

Mainly excreted in the urine as metabolites (consider dose reduction if renal impairment)

Storage

Available as 2 mg and 5 mg tablets or 100 mg vial for injection with diluent. Stable for 24 hours after reconstitution. Tablets and injection stored away from direct sunlight at room temperature

Mercaptopurine (6-MP, Puri-Nethol)

Group: antimetabolite

Dosage

50–75 mg/m^2 orally daily continuous treatment

Administration

Orally, 50 mg tablet

Precautions

Allopurinol blocks metabolism. Stop this drug when possible or reduce dose of mercaptopurine by 75%

Toxicity

+ + + Myelosuppression
+ Nausea and vomiting
Liver dysfunction
Mucositis
Skin rash

Monitoring tests

Full blood count, liver function tests, check if patient is taking allopurinol

5 Anticancer drugs

5.1 Alphabetical list of cytotoxic and hormonal agents

Metabolism and excretion

> Oxidation in liver to inactive form; 50% excreted in the urine in 24 hours (consider dose reduction for renal impairment)

Storage

> Tablets stable at room temperature

Interactions

> Allopurinol

Methotrexate (Emtexate, Maxtrex)

Group: antimetabolite

Dosage

> Multiple treatment schedules are in use
> Consult manufacturers' literature and clinical data
> Intrathecal, 5.0–12.5 mg once or twice weekly

Precautions

> Modify dose or omit if renal impairment
> Folinic acid rescue must be given if dose >200 mg/m^2 (see folinic acid, p. 142)
> May accumulate in effusions and cause prolonged toxicity. High dose contraindicated in this setting

Administration

> Orally, 2.5 mg, 10 mg tablets
> i.v. bolus + N. saline flush or infusion
> Intrathecal (see section 5.10)
> Intracavitary (see section 5.12)

Toxicity

> + + + Myelosuppression (nadir at 7–10 days, recovery at 14–16 days)
> Mucositis
> Nausea and vomiting (high dose)
> + + Diarrhoea
> Skin rash
> Cerebral atrophy

5.1   Alphabetical list of cytotoxic and hormonal agents

Renal dysfunction (high dose)
+ Alopecia
Pneumonitis
Malabsorption
Ocular
Liver dysfunction
Osteoporosis

Monitoring tests

Full blood count, liver function test, renal function; methotrexate levels if using high dose

Metabolism and excretion

75% excreted unchanged in urine in first 5 hours. Consider dose reduction if renal impairment and only use high dose if renal function normal

Storage

Tablets — room temperature
Solution — 5, 50, 500, 1000 and 5000 mg vials, room temperature
Opened vials — refrigerated, 24 hours

Interactions

5-fluorouracil, alcohol, aspirin, corticosteroids, hypo-glycaemic agents, probenecid, sulphonamides

Mitomycin (Mitomycin C Kyowa)

Group: antibiotic

Dosage

Consult clinical and pharmaceutical literature

Administration

i.v. bolus + N. saline flush

Precautions

May cause severe phlebitis and pain at the site of injection
Prolonged myelosuppression

5.1   Alphabetical list of cytotoxic and hormonal agents

Toxicity

+++ Myelosuppression (nadir at 3–4 weeks; recovery by 6–8 weeks)

Phlebitis and pain

++ Nausea and vomiting

Anorexia

Mucositis

Diarrhoea

Alopecia

Monitoring tests

Full blood count and renal function

Metabolism and excretion

Metabolized primarily in the liver

About 10% excreted unchanged in the urine

Storage

Powder — 2, 10 and 20 mg vials, room temperature

Solution — only stable for a few minutes

Mitotane* (op-DDD)

Group: hormonal agent, anti-adrenal
Dosage

1.0–2.5 g q.d.s., continuously

Administration

Orally, 500 mg tablets

Precautions

Steroid replacement if total dose more than 3 g/day

Discontinue in the event of intercurrent infection, trauma, etc.

Toxicity

++++ Nausea and vomiting

Adrenal insufficiency (ensure adequate replacement)

++ Sedation

Monitoring tests

Urea and electrolytes, lying and standing BP

5.1   Alphabetical list of cytotoxic and hormonal agents

Metabolism and excretion

> Excretion in the urine as metabolites. Urinary metabolites detectable for many months

Storage

> Room temperature

Mitozantrone (Novantrone)

Group: miscellaneous

Dosage

> 8–14 mg/m^2 i.v. every 3 weeks
>
> Multiple other schedules in use

Administration

> Short term i.v. infusion. Avoid in presence of cardiac disease. Monitor cardiac function if total dose exceeds 160 mg/m^2

Precautions

> Avoid contact with skin or eyes

Toxicity

+ + + Myelosuppression

+ + Mucositis

> Nausea and vomiting
>
> Alopecia
>
> Tissue necrosis
>
> Cardiomyopathy
>
> May impart blue–green coloration to urine 24 hours after administration

Monitoring tests

> Full blood count. Care if total dose >160 mg/m^2. Cardiac monitoring recommended if higher dose used (e.g. radionuclide ejection fraction). Monitor at lower doses if cardiac disease or previous Adriamycin

Metabolism and excretion

> Hepatic metabolism and hepatic and bilary excretion

151

5.1 Alphabetical list of cytotoxic and hormonal agents

Storage

> 20, 25 and 30 mg vials. Store at room temperature.
> Once diluted use within 24 hours

Mustine (mechlorethamine, HN_2, nitrogen mustard)

Group: alkylating agent
Dosage

> $2-6$ mg/m^2 i.v. every $3-4$ weeks
> $0.2-0.25$ mg/ml topically

Administration

> i.v. bolus into fast-running N. saline infusion
> Topically (see section 5.11)

Precautions

> Avoid extravasation
> Avoid contact with skin and eyes (wear gloves and
> goggles when preparing and injecting)

Toxicity

$+ + + +$ Tissue necrosis if extravasated
> Phlebitis
> Nausea and vomiting

$+ + +$ Myelosuppression (nadir at $9-14$ days;
> recovery at $16-20$ days)
> Alopecia

$+$ Pulmonary fibrosis
> Leukaemogenic

Monitoring tests

> Full blood count

Metabolism and excretion

> Inactive metabolites excreted in the urine

Storage

> Powder — 10 mg vials refrigerated
> Solution — only stable for a few minutes

5   Anticancer drugs

5.1   Alphabetical list of cytotoxic and hormonal agents

Oestrogens

Group: hormonal agents

Drugs, dosage and administration

        stilboestrol (1 mg and 5 mg tablets)

          breast carcinoma: 10–20 mg/day orally

          prostatic carcinoma: 1–3 mg/day orally

        ethinyloestradiol (1 mg tablets)

          1–3 mg/day, orally, i.m.

        polyoestradiol phosphate (Estradurin, 40 mg vial)

          prostatic carcinoma: 40–80 mg every 2–4 weeks, i.m.

Precautions

        Use with care in patients with heart failure

Metabolism

        Liver

Toxicity

  + + + + Feminization (e.g. gynaecomastia)

    + + + Fluid retention

        Hypertension

        Nausea and vomiting

      + + Thrombosis

Storage

        See manufacturers' literature for individual drugs

Plicamycin (Mithracin, mithramycin)

Group: antibiotic

Dosage

        Hypercalcaemia: 25 µg/kg, daily for 3–4 days, every
        10–14 days

Administration

        i.v. infusion over 4–6 hours

Toxicity

    + + + Nausea and vomiting

        Hypocalcaemia

+ + Phlebitis
Pyrexia
Coagulopathy
Myelosuppression
Drowsiness
+ Hepatic

Monitoring tests

Full blood count, calcium, coagulation screen if indicated

Metabolism and excretion

40% excreted in the urine within 15 hours

Consider dose reduction if renal function impaired

Storage

Powder — 2.5 mg vials, refrigerated

Solution — only stable for a few minutes

Procarbazine (Natulan)

Group: miscellaneous

Dosage

In combinations, 100 mg/m^2 daily $\times$ 14, every 4 weeks

Administration

Orally, 50 mg capsule

Precautions

Avoid tyramine-containing foods because of weak MAO inhibition

Toxicity

+ + + + Myelosuppression
+ + Nausea and vomiting (initially but less as therapy continues)
Rash
+ Mucositis
Pulmonary fibrosis
Encephalopathy
Leukaemogenic

5 Anticancer drugs

5.1 Alphabetical list of cytotoxic and hormonal agents

Metabolism and excretion
> Liver and renal clearance

Storage
> Room temperature

Monitoring tests
> Full blood count

Interactions
> Tyramine-containing foods, antihistamines, alcohol, hypoglycaemic agents

Progestogens

Group: hormonal agents
Drugs, dosage and administration
> *medroxyprogesterone acetate* (Farlutal, Provera, 100, 200, 250, 400 and 500 mg tablets)
>> 200–400 mg/day orally,
>> Depo-Provera 450 mg vial
>
> *gestronol hexanoate* (Depostat, 200 mg amp.)
>> 200–400 mg/week, i.m.
>
> *hydroxyprogesterone hexanoate*
> (Proluton depot, 250 mg and 500 mg syringes)
>> 1 g/week, i.m.
>
> *megestrol acetate* (Megace, 40 mg tabs)
>> 80–320 mg/day, orally

Precautions
> Ensure i.m. injections not given i.v. or s.c. Reduce dose if liver disease

Toxicity
> ++ Fluid retention, sterile abscesses (i.m. route)

Metabolism
> Liver

Storage
> See manufacturers' literature for individual drugs

5   Anticancer drugs

5.1   Alphabetical list of cytotoxic and hormonal agents

Razoxane (Razoxin, ICRF 159)

Group: miscellaneous
Dosage
> Consult manufacturers' literature

Administration
> Orally, 125 mg tablets

Precautions
> Nil specific

Toxicity
> + + +   Myelosuppression (nadir at 2 weeks; recovery by 3 weeks)
>
> Alopecia
>
> + +   Nausea and vomiting
>
> Diarrhoea
>
> Leukaemogenic
>
> +   Mucositis
>
> Acneiform rash

Monitoring tests
> Full blood count

Metabolism and excretion
> Liver and renal clearance

Storage
> Room temperature, 2 years

Streptozotocin (Streptozocin)

Group: nitrosourea
Dosage
> 1.0–1.5 g/m^2 weekly $\times$ 4 — repeat at 8 weeks, or
> 0.5–1.0 g/m^2 daily $\times$ 5 — repeat every 4–6 weeks

Administration
> i.v. infusion in 100–250 mg 5% dextrose over 10–15 min

5.1   Alphabetical list of cytotoxic and hormonal agents

i.v. infusion in 500 ml 5% dextrose over 6 hours

i.v. bolus

Precautions

Avoid extravasation

Acute hypoglycaemia can be induced by release of insulin from damaged islet cells, especially in treatment of insulinoma

Ensure adequate hydration

Toxicity

$+ + + +$ Tissue necrosis

$+ + +$ Nausea and vomiting

Renal failure (may be a transient rise in blood urea, or tubule damage and Fanconi's syndrome)

$+ +$ Phlebitis (pain at injection site with too rapid infusion)

Myelosuppression (mainly anaemia)

Hypoglycaemia (see above)

$+$ Hyperglycaemia (may occur after long-term use)

Metabolism and excretion

Liver metabolism and renal clearance

Storage

Refrigerated, 3 years

Monitoring tests

Full blood count, urea and electrolytes, blood and urine glucose

Interactions

Phenytoin

Tamoxifen (Nolvadex, Noltam, Tamofen)

Group: hormonal agent, anti-oestrogen

Dosage

20 mg daily, continuously

Administration

Orally, 10 and 20 mg tablets

5   Anticancer drugs

5.1   Alphabetical list of cytotoxic and hormonal agents

Precautions
>   Avoid during pregnancy

Toxicity
>   +++ Menopausal symptoms
>   + Nausea and vomiting
>   Thrombocytopenia (transient)

Metabolism and excretion
>   Probable enterophepatic circulation of metabolites

Storage
>   Room temperature, avoid light

Thioguanine (6-TG, 6-thioguanine, Lanvis)

Group: antimetabolite

Dosage
>   100 mg/m^2 orally, twice daily

Administration
>   Orally, 40 mg tablets

Precaution
>   Reduce dose if abnormal liver or renal function

Toxicity
>   +++ Myelosuppression (nadir 10–12 days; recovery 16–18
>   days)
>   ++ Diarrhoea
>   Nausea and vomiting
>   Liver toxicity (consider dose reduction if liver function
>   abnormal)

Monitoring tests
>   Full blood count and liver and renal function tests

Metabolism and excretion
>   Rapidly enters purine pathways
>   Metabolites excreted primarily via the kidney

Storage
>   Solution — refrigerated, 24 hours

5.1   Alphabetical list of cytotoxic and hormonal agents

Thiotepa (triethylenethiophosphoramide)

Group: alkylating agent

Dosage
>   See manufacturers' and clinical literature

Administration
>   i.v. bolus + N. saline flush
>   i.m.
>   intracavitary
>   intrathecally (see section 5.10)

Toxicity
>   + + + Myelosuppression
>   Sterility
>   Amenorrhoea
>   + + Nausea and vomiting
>   + Local pain
>   Leukaemogenic

Monitoring tests
>   Full blood count

Metabolism and excretion
>   85% is excreted in the urine

Storage
>   Powder — 15 mg vials, refrigerated
>   Solution — refrigerated, stable for days

Interactions
>   Neuromuscular blockers

Treosulfan (L-threitol, 1, 4-dimethane sulphonate)

Group: alkylating agent

Dosage
>   1 g p.o. daily in divided doses, continuously for 1 month and then alternate months if used as a single agent

5.1   Alphabetical list of cytotoxic and hormonal agents

Administration
>   Injection — 5–15 g i.v. every 1–3 weeks
>   Orally — 250 mg capsules

Toxicity
>   +++ Myelosuppression (nadir after 2–3 weeks of each
>   course)
>   ++ Nausea and vomiting
>   + Abdominal pain
>   Skin rash
>   Alopecia
>   Stomatitis (especially if capsule chewed)
>   Leukaemogenic

Monitoring tests
>   Full blood count

Storage
>   Room temperature

Vinblastine (Velbe)

Group: vinca alkaloid

Dosage
>   6–10 mg/m^2

Administration
>   i.v. bolus in 10–20 ml N. saline + flush with N. saline

Precautions
>   Avoid extravasation

Toxicity
> ++++ Myelosuppression (moderate to severe: nadir at 1 week;
>   recovery 2–3 weeks)
>   +++ Tissue necrosis
>   Nausea and vomiting
>   Neuropathy
>   Phlebitis
>   ++ Constipation
>   Alopecia

+ SIADH
Muscle pain (especially jaw pain)
Mucositis
Monitoring tests
Full blood count
Storage
10 mg vial
Dry — refrigerated, away from light
Solution — refrigerated, away from light, 4 weeks
Metabolism and excretion
Liver and kidney

Vincristine (Oncovin)

Group: vinca alkaloid
Dosage
Adults: 0.4–1.4 mg/m^2 (maximum 2 mg or 1.5 mg if age >65 years)
Children: up to 2 mg/m^2
Administration
i.v. bolus in 10–20 ml N. saline + flush with N. saline
Precautions
Avoid extravasation
Toxicity
+ + + + Neuropathy (may be dose-limiting)
+ + + Tissue necrosis
Nausea and vomiting
Alopecia
Constipation (can be severe)
Phlebitis
+ + Muscle pain (especially jaw pain)
+ SIADH
Myelosuppression
Mucositis
Seizures

5.1   Alphabetical list of cytotoxic and hormonal agents

Monitoring tests
> Full blood count

Storage
> 1, 2 and 5 mg vials
> Dry — refrigerated, away from light, 6 months
> Solution — refrigerated, away from light, 2 weeks

Metabolism
> Liver and kidney

Interactions
> Isoniazid, pyridoxine

Vindesine (Eldisine)

Group: vinca alkaloid

Dosage
> Adults: 3–4 mg/m^2
> Children: 4–5 mg/m^2

Administration
> i.v. bolus in 10–20 ml N. saline + flush with N. saline

Precautions
> Avoid extravasation

Toxicity
+ + + + Myelosuppression (moderate to severe: nadir at day 3–5; recovery by day 6–8)
  + + + Tissue necrosis
> Neuropathy
> Alopecia
> Phlebitis

    + + Constipation
> Nausea and vomiting

Storage
> Dry — refrigerated, 1–2 years
> Solution — refrigerated, 2 weeks

Metabolism and excretion
> Liver and kidney

Monitoring tests
>   Full blood count

5.2   Toxicity

Listed here, according to body systems, are the more common toxicities associated with cytotoxic drugs. This list is by no means comprehensive but is a guide to those likely to be encountered. If any unexpected toxicity occurs, reference should be made to the manufacturer's literature. Any new suspected toxicity should be reported to the Committee on Safety of Medicines, by yellow card.

The following scale of frequency is:

+ + + +   inevitable

+ + +   common

+ +   infrequent

+   rare

This can only be an approximate guide as many toxicities are dose dependent and, in combination, drugs may be synergistic in producing toxicity.

Cutaneous

Alopecia

+ + + +   Adriamycin, daunorubicin, epirubicin

+ + +   bleomycin, cyclophosphamide, etoposide, ifosfamide, mustine, razoxane

+ +   amsacrine, lomustine, mitomycin, mitozantrone, teniposide, vinblastine, vincristine, vindesine

+   actinomycin D, fluorouracil, mercaptopurine, methotrexate, treosulfan

Pigmentation

+ + + +   bleomycin

+ + +   Adriamycin, alkylating agents, 5-fluorouracil

+ +   actinomycin D, fluorouracil (especially high dose)

+   hydroxyurea

163

5.2   Toxicity

Rash (all cytotoxic drugs can be associated with allergic rashes but
the most common are given here)
+++ aminoglutethimide
++ procarbazine, chlorambucil

Tissue necrosis (on extravasation)
++++ actinomycin, Adriamycin, amsacrine, carmustine,
       daunorubicin, epirubicin, mustine, streptozotocin
+++ vinblastine, vincristine, vindesine
++ dacarbazine

Hyperkeratosis
+++ bleomycin

Nail changes (pigmentation, ridging, onycholysis)
+++ Adriamycin, bleomycin, cyclophosphamide
++ Fluorouracil, melphalan
+ hydroxyurea

Gastrointestinal

Mucositis
+++ actinomycin, Adriamycin, amsacrine, daunorubicin,
       epirubicin, methotrexate (especially high dose)
++ bleomycin, cytarabine, fluorouracil, lomustine, mercapto-
       purine, plicamycin
+ cyclophosphamide, hydroxyurea, melphalan, mitomycin,
       procarbazine, thioguanine, treosulfan, vinblastine,
       vincristine, razoxane

Nausea and vomiting
++++ carmustine, cisplatin, dacarbazine, mitotane, mustine
+++ actinomycin, Adriamycin, amsacrine, androgens, car-
       boplatin, cyclophosphamide, daunorubicin, epirubicin,
       etoposide (oral), hexamethylmelamine, hydroxyurea,

ifosfamide, lomustine, mithramycin, methotrexate (high dose), oestrogens, streptozotocin, vinblastine, vincristine

++ asparaginase, cytarabine, etoposide, fluorouracil, mercaptopurine, melphalan, mitomycin, procarbazine, razoxane, teniposide, thioguanine, thiotepa, treosulfan, vindesine

+ bleomycin, busulphan, chlorambucil, tamoxifen

Peptic ulcer

++ glucocorticoids

Malabsorption

+ fluorouracil, methotrexate

Diarrhoea

+++ cisplatin

++ cytarabine, fluorouracil, methotrexate (especially high dose), mitomycin, razoxane, thioguanine

Constipation

+++ vinblastine, vincristine

++ vindesine

Hepatic

+++ asparaginase

++ androgens, carmustine, mercaptopurine, methotrexate

+ chlorambucil, plicamycin

Abdominal pain

++ vincristine, vinblastine

+ fluorouracil, treosulfan

5 Anticancer drugs

5.2 Toxicity

Pulmonary

Lung infiltrates/fibrosis
+++ bleomycin
+ busulphan, chlorambucil, cyclophosphamide, lomustine, methotrexate, mustine, procarbazine

Cardiovascular

Phlebitis (at injection site)
++++ actinomycin, Adriamycin, amsacrine, carmustine, epirubicin, mustine
+++ dacarbazine, daunorubicin, ifosfamide, mitomycin, vinblastine, vincristine, vindesine
++ fluorouracil, plicamycin, streptozotocin
+ bleomycin

Raynaud's phenomenon
++ cisplatin, bleomycin in combination

Cardiomyopathy
++++ Adriamycin, daunorubicin, epirubicin, mitozantrone
++ cyclophosphamide (high dose)

Hypotension
++ etoposide (rapid i.v. injection)
+ aminoglutethimide, mitotane (if inadequate steroid replacement)

Fluid retention
+++ corticosteroids, progestogens, oestrogens

5   Anticancer drugs

5.2   Toxicity

Urogenital

Renal failure
- +++ streptozotocin
- ++ cisplatin (adequate hydration and avoid aminoglycoside antibiotics and loop diuretics)
- ++ methotrexate (high dose — ensure adequate renal function, alkalinize urine and folinic acid rescue; see section 5.6)
- + asparaginase, ifosfamide, thioguanine

Haemorrhagic cystitis
- ++++ ifosfamide (give mesna; see section 5.8)
- +++ cyclophosphamide (see section 5.8)
- + melphalan

Infertility (see section 5.3)
- +++ alkylating agents, procarbazine

Neuromuscular

Encephalopathy
- +++ asparaginase, ifosfamide
- + procarbazine

Cerebral atrophy (see section 5.3)
- ++ methotrexate (especially with cranial irradiation)

Seizures
- ++ cisplatin
- + vincristine

Cerebellar syndrome
- + fluorouracil

5   Anticancer drugs

5.2   Toxicity

Neuropathy
+ + + + vincristine
+ + + vinblastine, vindesine
+ + cisplatin

Ototoxicity
+ + + cisplatin

Sedation
+ + + aminoglutethimide
+ + plicamycin, mitotane, ifosfamide

Muscle pain
+ + vincristine
+ vinblastine

Endocrine/metabolic

Adrenal insufficiency
+ + + + glucocorticoids, mitotane
+ + + aminoglutethimide

Inappropriate ADH secretion
+ cyclophosphamide, vinblastine, vincristine

Hypocalcaemia
+ + + plicamycin
+ + cisplatin (rarely symptomatic)

Hypomagnesaemia
+ + + cisplatin (common biochemically, rarely symptomatic)

Hyperglycaemia
+ + + asparaginase, glucocorticoids
+ + streptozotocin (long term)

5.2   Toxicity

Hypoglycaemia
+ + streptozotocin (acute)

Hypoalbuminaemia
+ asparaginase

Haematological
Marrow depression (almost all cytotoxic drugs cause some degree
of depression, except vincristine, bleomycin and asparaginase. See
individual drugs for frequency, severity, and time to recovery).

Coagulopathy
+ + plicamycin

Hypofibrinogenaemia
+ asparaginase

Ocular

Dry eyes/conjunctivitis
+ fluorouracil, methotrexate

Lacrimation
+ fluorouracil, methotrexate, Adriamycin

Increased intraocular pressure
+ + + corticosteroids

Papillitis
+ cisplatin

Cataract
+ + corticosteroids
+ busulphan

5.2   Toxicity

Pyrexia/rigors

+ + + asparaginase, bleomycin

+ + Adriamycin, dacarbazine, plicamycin

Second tumours (see section 5.3)

5.3   Long-term problems

When there is a high chance of prolonged survival following chemotherapy, long-term problems become more important. They should particularly be considered when adjuvant chemotherapy is planned because, inevitably, a percentage of patients will be receiving 'unnecessary' treatment. In the case of life-threatening but chemo-sensitive tumours (e.g. Hodgkin's disease and testicular teratoma), complete remission is the first priority and only when regimens of equal efficacy have been established, can one afford the luxury of selecting treatment because of lesser long-term toxicity.

Male sexual function

A number of cytotoxic drugs, in particular the alkylating agents, cause azoospermia. The duration of this following treatment and the completeness of recovery depend on the dose and duration of the treatment. However, the majority of men who have received alkylating agents in combination with other drugs for Hodgkin's disease for at least 6 courses, are rendered permanently sterile. Other drugs have less of an effect and there are now a number of reports of men who have produced children after receiving cisplatin-containing combination chemotherapy for testicular teratoma.

Although there is a theoretical risk of teratogenic effects on germ cells, this has not in practice proved to be a problem. There is no increased risk of birth defects in children conceived after chemotherapy is stopped.

Leydig cell function in adults seems to be affected only slightly if at all and testosterone levels are usually maintained.

Sperm banking should be considered for men receiving chemotherapy with alkylating agents who might subsequently wish to father children. However, it has been found that many men with Hodgkin's disease, especially those with systemic symptoms, have low sperm counts or inactive spermatozoa before starting treatment. Similarly, testicular teratoma is often associated with subfertility and changes in the other testicle. In such cases, sperm banking is not worthwhile.

Impotence is a common problem during chemotherapy but almost always has an emotional and psychological cause. Failure to ejaculate, despite normal potency and orgasm, often occurs in men who have undergone retroperitoneal lymphadenectomy.

Female sexual function

Amenorrhoea is very common in women receiving anticancer drugs, especially alkylating agents. Recovery depends on the dose and duration of chemotherapy, as well as on the age of the patient. Menstruation is unlikely to return in women over 30-35 years old who have received a significant amount of treatment, whereas it usually does in younger patients. Girls treated before puberty almost all develop normally (for pregnancy and contraception see section 4.11). Hormone replacement should be given to young women who develop amenorrhoea after chemotherapy. There is *no* good evidence for long-term teratogenic effects on germ cells or increased risk of birth defects in children conceived after chemotherapy is stopped.

Growth retardation

High-dose corticosteroid therapy, such as is given with many chemotherapy regimens for lymphoid malignancy and leukaemia, may retard growth and should be kept to a minimum in children.

Cerebral atrophy

Cerebral atrophy and mild impairment of intellectual function has been noted in children who have received combinations of high-dose and intrathecal methotrexate and cerebral irradiation in the treatment of leukaemia.

5.3   Long-term problems

Second tumours

As more patients have survived following chemotherapy, a marked increase in the number of second tumours recorded has been noted, some of which may be treatment-related. In animal studies, alkylating agents, some antitumour antibiotics and procarbazine, seem to be the most carcinogenic, whereas antimetabolites seem relatively innocuous in this respect. The most important clinical problem is the development of acute leukaemia (usually undifferentiated or myelogenous). In patients treated successfully for Hodgkin's disease, the incidence is as high as 1% per year in patients who have received both radiotherapy and chemotherapy, such as MOPP. Similar second tumours have also been reported following long-term alkylating agent therapy for ovarian carcinoma.

5.4   Intravenous drug administration

Many cytotoxic drugs are given intravenously, for several reasons:

1   The drug is not absorbed from the gastrointestinal tract.

2   The drug is too irritating to the gastrointestinal tract.

3   The drug is unstable and may coagulate tissue proteins, if given i.m.

4   Higher drug levels can be obtained.

5   The drug has a narrow therapeutic ratio and so accurate blood levels are important.

6   Compliance is not a problem.

Because many cytotoxic drugs cause phlebitis and most patients require multiple courses of drugs in addition to blood transfusions and perhaps intravenous fluids and antibiotics, care of veins and techniques of intravenous therapy are very important. Many hospitals have *trained specialist chemotherapy nurses* who give all the treatment. Such nurses not only become expert at intravenous injections but can spend time explaining the details of complex regimens and giving the patients advice on preventing and coping with toxicities.

The technique for setting up the intravenous infusion or injection is the same as for other i.v. treatments but some points are worth emphasizing:

5   Anticancer drugs

5.4   Intravenous drug administration

1   Find the right vein: use a sphygmomanometer cuff rather than a tourniquet because it gives better control; immerse the patient's arm in hot water for 5–10 min if no veins are easily seen; use veins in the following order of preference: forearm, dorsum of hand, wrist, antecubital fossa; use large-bore veins if possible when an irritant drug is to be given; never use leg or foot veins.

2   Use the right cannula: 21 gauge or 23 gauge steel 'butterfly' for bolus or short infusions; plastic cannula for long infusions.

3   Ensure the cannula is in the vein: draw back 1–2 ml of blood; give test injection of 1–2 ml N. saline.

4   Inject slowly: watch for signs of extravasation, ask patient to report pain at injection site; do not force the injection if there is apparent resistance.

5   Flush: follow all injections with a flush of 5–10 ml of N. saline.

Irritants

The following drugs may cause local irritation of veins:

- Adriamycin
- actinomycin D
- amsacrine
- carmustine
- dacarbazine
- daunorubicin
- epirubicin
- mitomycin C
- mustine
- vinblastine
- vincristine
- vindesine

These drugs should not be injected directly into veins but into the side arm of a fast-flowing drip. They should be injected slowly (c. 5–10 ml/min) and not allowed to 'back up' into the infusion line, giving a high concentration. Watch carefully for extravasation and ask the patient about pain at the injection site. All these drugs may cause temporary venous spasm, reddening of the skin over the vein or pain along the course of the vein, without extravasating. If any of

173

5.4   Intravenous drug administration

these occur, stop the injection and allow the saline infusion to run for a minute or so until the symptoms subside. If in any doubt, resite the cannula.

Alternatives

In patients who are about to have a prolonged course of intravenous treatment, such as adults with acute myelogenous leukaemia or in those with veins already damaged by treatment, long intravenous catheters may be considered. Recently, a number of centres have started to use the 'Hickman' or other comparable catheters. These are special catheters introduced into the cephalic or subclavian vein. The external part of the catheter is 'tunnelled' for a short distance under the skin to reduce the risk of infection. Provided the exit site is carefully cleaned every day and flushed out with heparin, such a line can be kept in for several months and used for:

• all blood taking and transfusions
• all chemotherapy administration
• antibiotic therapy
• parenteral nutrition

Patients and their families can usually be taught to care for the line and it can be used in outpatients. It is a useful alternative in patients who are about to embark on a prolonged course of treatment, in whom it is best implanted before treatment starts.

A minor operation is needed to place the catheter. The main complications are infection and thrombosis.

5.5   Prevention and treatment of drug extravasation

Despite great care, local tissue reactions occur and account for up to 5% of all adverse effects of anticancer drugs. There are a number of factors which increase the risk of a significant local tissue effect:

1   Some drugs are much more irritant than others. Table 5.1 shows the likely tissue effects of many of the commonly used drugs.

2   The degree of dilution of the drug and amount extravasated.

3   The site of injection. Injections in the antecubital fossa should be

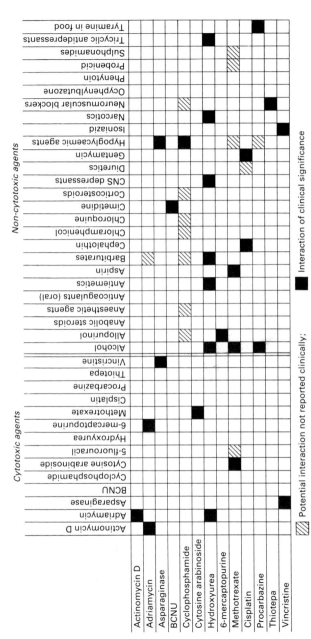

Table 5.1. Drug interactions of cytotoxic drugs (adapted from J. Stuart and I. Stockley). Some of these interactions are theoretical and have only been demonstrated in animal models.

■ Interaction of clinical significance; ▨ Potential interaction not reported clinically

avoided as extravasation is more difficult to detect in this area and slough may expose nerves and tendons, resulting in permanent dysfunction. Extravasation over the back of the hand is also particularly morbid.

4   Old and debilitated patients, often with vascular disease, seem more prone to this toxicity.

5   Patients with venous obstruction (most common superior vena cava obstruction) are at particular risk and it is best to try to avoid using vesicant drugs in these patients.

6   Previous irradiation to the site of extravasation increases the risk of a severe reaction.

7   Extravasation into an arm whose lymphatic drainage has been impaired (by surgery, radiotherapy or axillary node involvement), also increases the risk of a severe reaction.

Treatment
There have been no controlled studies that have compared regimens for the treatment of this complication. Treatment should be started immediately and recommendations include the following:

1   Stop the injection immediately but *do not* remove the needle.

2   Using the needle, withdraw 3–5 ml of blood in an attempt to remove the drug.

3   Using a fine (27 gauge) needle or a Tine (TB) syringe, aspirate the subcutaneous tissue to remove as much drug as possible.

4   Remove the needle.

5   Elevate the arm and apply ice packs to the extravasation site 4 times daily for 3 days. No proven antidote exists and it is recommended that *no* local drug injections are given.

6   If pain persists or vesiculation or ulceration occur seek advice from a plastic surgeon.

5.6   Administration of high-dose methotrexate
High-dose methotrexate (>200 mg/m^2) is potentially dangerous and its therapeutic value often unproven. It should *only* be used by those experienced in medical oncology.

5   Anticancer drugs

5.6   Administration of high-dose methotrexate

The toxic effects of very high doses of methotrexate can be prevented if folinic acid 'rescue' is given within 48 hours of treatment. There are numerous regimens for the administration of methotrexate in this fashion but there are several important factors if it is to be done safely:

1   This treatment should be avoided in the presence of ascites, pleural effusion or oedema.

2   The patient must have normal renal function before treatment.

3   The urine must be alkalinized to prevent crystallinuria.

4   The drugs must be given with and followed by an intravenous infusion.

5   If doses of more than $1 \ g/m^2$ are used, then plasma methotrexate levels should be monitored.

6   Folinic acid is usually started at 24 hours and the dose and duration of 'rescue' should ideally be dictated by the plasma methotrexate level.

7   Renal function should be monitored — a worsening creatinine indicates the need for prolonged rescue.

Alkalinization of the urine is achieved as follows:

1   Give acetozolamide 250 mg the night before treatment and continue for 2 further days.

2   Give 500 ml 1.4% sodium bicarbonate and 500 ml dextrose-saline, over 2 hours, prior to the methotrexate.

3   Check that the urine pH is greater than 7.0.

4   Infuse methotrexate (1–4 hours) in 500–1000 ml of N. saline.

5   Continue intravenous fluids dextrose-saline (with or without potassium) 1 litre/6 hours.

6   Check urine pH hourly — if less than 7.0, give further sodium bicarbonate.

5.7   Pre-hydration regimen for cisplatin

Unless cisplatin is given with a large fluid load, it is nephrotoxic. Because of the need for prolonged intravenous infusion and the nausea and vomiting caused by cisplatin, most patients have to be admitted to hospital for their chemotherapy. Outpatient regimens can be used safely but many patients prefer hospital admission because of the severe emesis.

Inpatient regimen

1   Start infusion of normal saline with 10 mmol of potassium chloride per litre. Give 500 ml per hour.

2   When urine output is greater than 200 ml/hour, give cisplatin as a bolus or short infusion. The use of mannitol is usually not necessary, unless there is evidence of fluid overload.

3   Continue i.v. infusion with N. saline or dextrose-saline, with or without potassium supplements, as indicated by pre-treatment electrolytes. The infusion should be given at a rate of 250 ml per hour. This infusion should last a minimum of 6 hours or until the patient stops vomiting.

Outpatient regimen

1   Start a 2-hour i.v. infusion of 2 litres of dextrose-saline with 10 mmol of KCl/litre.

2   Give frusemide 40 mg at the start of the infusion.

3   After 30 min, give 12.5 g of mannitol i.v.

4   Then give the cisplatin by a bolus.

5   If a brisk diuresis has not been produced by the frusemide, this should be repeated together with mannitol, until a diuresis of greater than 250 ml is achieved in the 30 min before the cisplatin is given.

5.8   Cystitis related to cyclophosphamide or ifosfamide

A chemical cystitis, characterized by frequency, dysuria and haematuria, is a relatively common problem in patients being treated with cyclophosphamide and is almost universal in those receiving ifosfamide. This cystitis is usually transient and not severe but, if the drugs are continued, severe problems can result. Serious persistent haematuria has been reported and total cystectomy has been necessary in a few cases.

Prevention is, therefore, important. The cystitis is caused by metabolic breakdown products (principally acrolein), accumulating at high concentration in the bladder. This can be prevented in two ways:

1   By maintaining a high fluid intake (at least 2 litres a day). This is often adequate in patients treated with cyclophosphamide.

2   By using a sulphydryl-containing compound (mesna) to inactivate the acrolein. This is essential in patients receiving high dose (>2 g i.v.) cyclophosphamide or ifosfamide at any dose.

Mesna is a new agent that has little tissue penetration and which is rapidly excreted in the urine. Pharmacokinetic studies do not appear to show any effect of mesna on the plasma decay curve of ifosfamide. Consult the pharmaceutical literature for details of administration.

5.9   Oral administration

Most cytotoxic drugs are given by injection, either because they are poorly absorbed from the gastrointestinal tract or because they produce too much local toxicity to be given by mouth. There are, however, a number that can be given orally and some that are formulated for oral use only.

Disadvantages
- the drug may be irritant to the gastric mucosa and induce nausea
- variable absorption
- lower peak levels
- uncertain patient compliance, especially if the drugs have an unpleasant taste or cause nausea

Advantages
- fewer hospital attendances
- fewer venepunctures
- suitable for chronic low-dose administration
- some side-effects (e.g. nausea) may be minimized by dividing doses.

5 Anticancer drugs

5.9 Oral administration

Special precautions
1 Nausea and local irritation can be minimized by taking drugs on a full stomach or at bed time.
2 Lomustine must be taken on an empty stomach.
3 Treosulfan capsules must be swallowed whole and not chewed, as they may cause stomatitis.
4 Patients on procarbazine must avoid tyramine-containing foods (e.g. cheese, red wine, meat extract), because of its weak MAO-inhibitory action.
5 If oral cytotoxic drugs are given for short courses rather than continuously, it is essential to specify clearly the number of days for which they are to be given, on prescriptions and letters to the family practitioner. In general, it is best that these drugs are dispensed only from hospital pharmacies.

5.10 Intrathecal administration
In general, cytotoxic drugs do not cross the intact blood–brain barrier (nitrosoureas and high-dose methotrexate being exceptions) but high cerebrospinal fluid (CSF) levels of certain drugs can be achieved by intrathecal administration. It is believed that such drugs injected into the CSF will circulate throughout the subarachnoid space. This is partly confirmed by tracer studies but intrathecal treatment if often combined with cranial or cranio-spinal irradiation, because of uncertainty about the efficiency of this circulation.

Indications for intrathecal chemotherapy are:
• proven involvement of the meninges with tumour
• prophylaxis against central nervous system (CNS) relapse in acute lymphoblastic leukaemia and some high-risk lymphomas

The following drugs can be given intrathecally:
1 Methotrexate, 5.0–12 mg twice weekly, until the CSF is clear of tumour cells.
2 Cytosine arabinoside, 50 mg twice weekly, until the CSF is clear of tumour cells. Dilute with sterile Ringer's lactate, Elliot's B solution or the patient's own CSF. The diluent provided for i.v. use must *not* be used.

3   Thiotepa, 1–10 mg twice weekly, until the CSF is clear of tumour cells. Dilute in sterile water for injection to a concentration of 1 mg/ml.

No other drugs can be used safely for intrathecal injection.

Lumbar puncture
1   Standard aseptic lumbar puncture (LP) procedure.
2   Remove a volume of CSF equal to volume to be injected (*c.* 10–15 ml).
3   Send CSF specimens for all relevant diagnostic investigations on the first occasion, and for bacteriology and cytology on all subsequent occasions.
4   Dilute the drug with CSF if necessary.
5   Ensure the needle is still in CSF and inject drug slowly.

Ommaya reservoir
In patients unable to tolerate frequent LPs, or if LP is technically difficult or when it is considered essential to deliver adequate doses of chemotherapy into the ventricles, an Ommaya reservoir with an intraventricular catheter can be implanted subcutaneously in the scalp.

The following procedure for drug instillation is used:
1   Keep scalp over reservoir shaved.
2   Aseptic technique.
3   Palpate reservoir and insert 21 gauge or 23 gauge needle.
Some models have a metal cup on the bottom to prevent puncturing both sides of the reservoir.
4   Aspirate suitable volume of CSF.
5   Inject drug.
6   Flush drug through by re-injecting aspirated CSF.

Complications
The following complications may be associated with intrathecal cytotoxic chemotherapy:
1   Headache and meningism.

5.10 Intrathecal administration

---

2   Marrow depression, especially following methotrexate intra-thecally in patients with poor bone marrow reserve.
3   Chemical arachnoiditis — plaeomorphic cell infiltrate in CSF.
4   Nausea and vomiting.
5   Infection — treat according to bacteriological findings. Infected Ommaya reservoirs should be removed.
6   Fever — if persistent, repeat LP to exclude infection.
7   Paraplegia and encephalopathy have been reported, following methotrexate and cytarabine. It may also occur when high doses are combined with irradiation.
8   Cerebral atrophy.

5.11 Topical administration

Only 2 cytotoxic drugs are used for topical application to skin lesions:
1   Fluorouracil, 5% cream, for treatment of superficial basal cell carcinoma and pre-malignant keratoses.
2   Mustine, 10–50% solution in normal saline, for treatment of superficial plaques of mycosis fungoides.

5.12 Intracavitary administration

Intrapleural

A number of drugs, both cytotoxic and other, can be used in the management of recurrent malignant pleural effusion. Pleural irritation and subsequent adhesion is, probably, the mechanism of action of most of those drugs.

The following can be used:
1   Tetracycline, 1 g — treatment of choice, because of minimal local and systemic side-effects.
2   Bleomycin, 30–90 mg — avoid high doses in patients with poor performance status or low albumin. May cause collapse and hypotension.
3   Thiotepa, 20–60 mg.

5.12 Intracavity administration

4 Mepacrin (quinacrine), 50–100 mg day 1, then 200 mg daily for 4 days, if tolerated.

5 Mustine — not recommended because of local pain, and marrow toxicity.

Technique

1 *Complete* aspiration of the effusion, preferably by tube drainage.

2 Dissolve drug in 100–150 ml of N. saline.

3 Instil into pleural cavity.

4 Remove tube or needle.

Intraperitoneal

Intraperitoneal instillation of drugs can be used in the management of recurrent malignant ascites but it is, generally, less successful than in the management of pleural effusion because:

- effectiveness depends on the antitumour, rather than the irritant effect of the drug
- the tumour may be resistant
- ascites may be multiloculated and the drug may not diffuse throughout the peritoneum

The following may be used:

- bleomycin, 30–90 mg. Avoid high doses in patients with poor performance status or low albumin — may cause collapse, and hypotension
- Thiotepa, 20–60 mg

Technique

1 Drain ascites as completely as possible over 12–24 hours.

2 Dissolve drug in 100–250 mg of N. saline.

3 Instil into peritoneal cavity and clamp off drain.

4 Vary patient's position over 6–8 hours to ensure distribution of drug.

5 Open tube and redrain for maximum of further 12 hours.

5.12 Intracavity administration

Intrapericardial

Although radiotherapy or systemic chemotherapy is the treatment of choice, drugs can be instilled into the pericardial cavity in the management of malignant effusion. The main function of the drugs is as an irritant to obliterate the pericardial space.

The following drugs have been used:

- tetracycline, 500 mg–1 g
- mepacrin, 50–100 mg for 5 days
- thiotepa, 45 mg

Appendices

1   Cancer chemotherapy regimens

This section is included to make it easy to refer to a number of commonly used regimens. Doctors who are not familiar with them or their indications should consult the original references. Space is left at the end of this section for the insertion of specific regimens.

ABVD (Hodgkin's disease)

Adriamycin	25 mg/m^2 i.v., days 1 + 14
Bleomycin	10 mg/m^2 i.v., days 1 + 14
Vinblastine	6 mg/m^2 (max. 10 mg) i.v., days 1 + 14
DTIC	350 mg/m^2 i.v., days 1 + 14
Cycle time	28 days (Bonnadonna *et al.*, 1975)

BEP (advanced teratoma and seminoma)

Bleomycin	30 mg i.v., days 2, 9 + 16
Etoposide	120 mg/m^2 i.v., days 1–3
Cisplatin	20 mg/m^2 i.v., days 1–5
Cycle time	21 days (Williams *et al.*, 1987)

CAV (small cell carcinoma of the bronchus)

Cyclophosphamide	1 g/m^2 i.v., day 1
Adriamycin	40 mg/m^2 i.v., day 1
Vincristine	1 mg/m^2 (max. 2 mg) i.v., day 1
Cycle time	21 days (Greco *et al.*, 1978)

ChIVPP (Hodgkin's disease)

Chlorambucil	6 mg/m^2 p.o., days 1–14
Vinblastine	6 mg/m^2 (max. 10 mg) i.v., days 1 + 8
Procarbazine	100 mg/m^2 p.o., days 1–14
Prednisolone	40 mg p.o., days 1–14
Cycle time	28 days (McElwain *et al.*, 1977)

CHOP (non-Hodgkin's lymphoma)

Cyclophosphamide	750 mg/m^2 i.v., day 1
Adriamycin	50 mg/m^2 i.v., day 1

1   Cancer chemotherapy regimens

Vincristine   1.4 mg/m^2 i.v. day 1 (max. 2 mg)
Prednisolone   50 mg/m^2 p.o. days 1–5
Cycle time   21 days (Armitage et al., 1982)

CMF (breast cancer)
Cyclophosphamide   100 mg/m^2 p.o., days 1–14
Methotrexate   40 mg/m^2 i.v., days 1 + 8
5-fluorouracil   600 mg/m^2 i.v., days 1 + 8
Cycle time   28 days (Canellos et al., 1976)

CVP (non-Hodgkin's lymphoma)
Cyclophosphamide   400 mg/m^2 p.o., days 1–5
Vincristine   1.4 mg/m^2 (max. 2 mg) i.v., day 1
Prednisolone   100 mg/m^2 p.o., days 1–5
Cycle time   21 days (Young et al., 1977)

MACOP-B (non-Hodgkin's lymphoma)
Methotrexate   400 mg/m^2 i.v., weeks 2,6,10
Adriamycin   50 mg/m^2 i.v., weeks 1,3,5,7,9,11
Cyclophosphamide   350 mg/m^2 i.v., weeks 1,3,5,7,9,11
Vincristine   1.4 mg/m^2 i.v., weeks 2,4,6,8,10,12
Bleomycin   10 mg/m^2 i.v., weeks 4,8,12
Prednisolone   75 mg p.o., daily
Total treatment period   12 weeks (Klimo and Connors, 1985)

MOPP (Hodgkin's disease)
Mustine   6 mg/m^2 i.v., days 1 + 8
Vincristine   1.4 mg/m^2 (max. 2 mg) i.v., days 1 + 8
Procarbazine   100 mg/m^2 p.o., days 1–14
Prednisolone   40 mg/m^2 p.o., days 1–14
Cycle time   28 days (Longo et al., 1986)

2   Body surface area nomogram

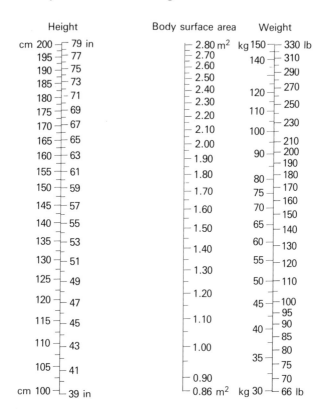

Nomogram for determination of body surface area from height and weight. From the formula of DuBois and DuBois (1916) $S = W^{0.425} \times H^{0.725} \times 71.84$, or log $S = W \times 0.425 + \log H \times 0.725 + 1.8564$, where S is body surface in cm^2, W is weight in kg and H is height in cm.

3   Gentamicin dosage nomogram

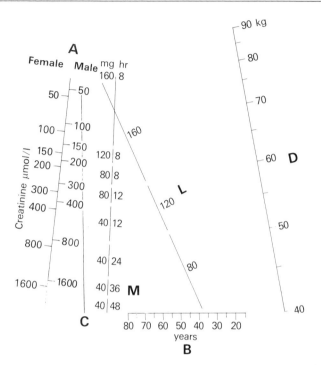

3   Gentamicin dosage nomogram

To determine a gentamicin dose schedule (Mawer, 1974)

1   Join with a straight line the serum creatinine concentration appropriate to the sex on scale A and the age on scale B. Mark the point at which the straight line cuts line C.

2   Join with a straight line the mark on line C and the body weight on scale D. Mark the points at which this line cuts the dosage lines L and M.

3   The loading dose (mg) is written against the marked part of line L. The maintenance dose (mg) and the appropriate interval

189

3   Gentamicin dosage nomogram

___

(hours) between the doses are written against the marked part of line M.

4 The nomogram is designed to give serum concentrations of gentamicin within the range 3–10 µg/ml, 2 hours after each dose. It is highly recommended that pre- and post-dose gentamicin levels are checked in all patients.

Example: male, serum creatinine 400 µmol/l, 45 years, 55 kg; loading dose 120 mg, maintenance dose 40 mg, 12–hourly.

4   Help agencies in cancer care in the UK

BACUP: British Association of Cancer United Patients and their families and friends. 121/123 Charterhouse Street, London EC1M 6AA. Cancer Information Service: Tel. 01-608 1661.

Department of Health and Social Security: grants and attendance allowances. Marie Curie Foundation Homes, Homes Department, 138 Sloane Street, London SW1X 9AY.

Hospice Care: available in all regions.

Ileostomy Association of Great Britain and Ireland, 149 Harley Street, London W1N 2DE.

Malcolm Sargent Fund for Children, Chief Administrator, 56 Redcliffe Square, London SW10.

Mastectomy Association, 1 Colworth Road, Croydon, Surrey CR0 7AD.

National Society for Cancer Relief, Sir Michael Sobell House, 30 Dorset Square, London NW1.

Red Cross: local branches provide aids and assistance.

Tenovus Cancer Information Centre, 111 Cathedral Road, Cardiff CF1 9PH.

5   Cancer research organizations

Cancer Research Campaign, 2 Carlton House Terrace, London SW1Y 5AR.

European Organization for Research on the Treatment of Cancer, Institut Jules Bordet, Rue Heger, Bordet 1, 1000, Bruxelles, Belgium.

Imperial Cancer Research Fund, Lincoln's Inn Fields, London WC2.

Leukaemia Research Fund, 43 Great Ormond Street, London WC1N 3JJ.

Medical Research Council, 20 Park Crescent, London W1N 48L.

National Cancer Institute, Westwood Building, Room 850, 5333 Westbard Avenue, Bethesda, Washington DC, USA.

United Kingdom Children's Cancer Study Group (UKCCSG), The Medical Statistics Department, The Christie Hospital and Holt Radium Institute, Withington, Manchester M20 9BX.

Regional cancer organizations in England and Wales

Northwestern RCO, Department of Social Research, Kinnaird Road, Manchester M20 9BX.

South West Thames RCO, Royal Marsden Hospital, Downs Road, Sutton, Surrey.

Wessex RCO, Royal South Hants Hospital, Southampton SO9 4YE.

Yorkshire RCO, Cookridge Hospital, Leeds LS16 6QB.

6   Books for patients

General

BACUP *Understanding Cancer Series*. 121/123 Charterhouse St., London EC1M 6AA.

Brody J. and Hollets A. (1977) *You can Fight Cancer and Win* New York, Times Book Inc.

Glucksberg H. and Singer J. (1979) *Cancer Care: a personal guide*. Baltimore, Johns Hopkins University Press.

Israel L. (1981) *Conquering Cancer*. London, Pelican.

Scott, Sir Ronald Bodley (1980) *Cancer: the facts*. Oxford, Oxford University Press.

US Department of Health and Human Services (1980) *Coping with Cancer*. National Cancer Institute, Bethesda, Maryland, USA.

Williams C.J. and William S. (1986) *Cancer: a guide for patients and their families*. Chichester, John Wiley.

Specific tumours

Baker L. (1978) *You and Leukaemia: a day at a time*. Philadelphia, Saunders.

Baum M. (1981) *Breast Cancer: the facts*. Oxford, Oxford University Press.

Cox B., Carr D. and Lee R. (1977) *Living with Lung Cancer: a reference book for people with lung cancer and their families*. Rochester, Schmidt Printing Inc.

Foulder C. (1979) *Breast Cancer*. London, Pan Books.

Newman J. (1976) What Every Woman Should Know About Breast Cancer. California, Major Books.

Williams C. J. (1984) *Lung Cancer: the facts*. Oxford, Oxford University Press.

See various associations in Appendix 4 for leaflets on specific tumours and other aspects of cancer.

Appendices

Notes

Appendices

Notes

Appendices

Notes

References and further reading

References
Armitage J.O. *et al.* (1982) *Cancer* **50**, 1695.
Bonnadonna G. *et al.* (1975) *Cancer* **36**, 252.
Canellos G.P. *et al.* (1976) *Cancer* **38**, 1882.
Carbone P.P. *et al.* (1971) *Cancer Res.* **31**, 1860.
DuBois and DuBois (1916) *Arch. Int. Med.* **17**, 863.
Durie B.G.M. and Salmon S.E. (1975) *Cancer* **36**, 842.
Greco F.A. *et al.* (1978) *Semin. Oncol.* **5**, 323.
Klimo P. and Connors J.M. (1985) *Ann. Int. Med.* **102**, 596.
Longo D. *et al.* (1986) *J. Clin. Oncol.* **4**, 1295.
Mawer G.E. *et al.* (1974) *Br. J. Clin. Pharm.* **1**, 45.
McElwain T.J. *et al.* (1977) *Br. J. Cancer* **36**, 276.
Peckham M.J. *et al.* (1979) *Lancet* **ii**, 267.
Rai K.R. *et al.* (1975) *Blood* **46**, 219.
Williams S.D. *et al.* (1987) *N. Engl. J. Med.* **316**, 1435.
Young R.C. *et al.* (1977) *Cancer Treat. Rep.* **61**, 1153.

Further reading
Calman K.C., Smyth J.F. and Tattersal M.H.N. (1980) *Basic Principles of Cancer Chemotherapy*. London, Macmillan.
de Vita V.T., Hellman S., Rosenberg S.A. (1987) *Cancer: Principles and Practices of Oncology*. Philadelphia, J.B. Lippincott.
Salmon S.E. and Jones S.E. (eds) (1981) *Adjuvant Therapy of Cancer III*. New York, Grune and Stratten.
Saunders C.M. (ed) (1978) *The Management of Terminal Disease*. London, Edward Arnold.
Selby P., McElwain T.J. (eds) (1987) *Hodgkin's Disease*. Oxford, Blackwell Scientific.
Seminars in Oncology. New York, Grune and Stratten.
Whitehouse J.M.A. and Mead G.M. (eds) (1985) *Early and Late Effects of Cancer Treatment*. London, Saunders.
Wilkes (ed) (1982) *The Dying Patient*. Lancaster, MTP Press Ltd.
Yarbro J.W. and Bornstein R.S. (1982) *Oncologic Emergencies*. New York, Grune and Stratten.

Index

Index